Essential Exercises for the Childbearing Year, 3rd edition
Having Twins, 2nd edition
Childbirth with Insight
Marie Osmond's Exercises for Mothers-to-be
Marie Osmond's Exercises for Mothers and Babies
Having Your Baby by Donor Insemination

Primal
Connections

ELIZABETH NOBLE

A FIRESIDE BOOK
PUBLISHED BY SIMON & SCHUSTER
NEW YORK   LONDON   TORONTO   SYDNEY
TOKYO   SINGAPORE

FIRESIDE
Simon & Schuster Building
Rockefeller Center
1230 Avenue of the Americas
New York, New York 10020

Designed by Chris Welch
Manufactured in the United States of America

10 9 8 7 6 5 4 3 2 1

Library of Congress Cataloging-in-Publication Data
Noble, Elizabeth, date
     Primal connections / Elizabeth Noble.
         p.   cm.
     "A fireside book."
     Includes bibliographical references and index.
     1. Prenatal influences. 2. Hypnotic age regression. 3. Primal
therapy. 4. Fetal behavior. I. Title.
RG635.N6   1993
155.2'34—dc20   92-29128
                                                              CIP

ISBN: 0-671-67851-5

To Julia and Carsten

My spirit guides whose enriching lives within me were such milestones in my ongoing journey of self-discovery.

Acknowledgments

The courageous people who took the risk to explore their inner domains are the lifeblood of this book, and I thank them for sharing their profound and intimate experiences so that light may shine on the various paths for others. I appreciate the many visionaries in the pre- and perinatal psychology movement, both in the USA and abroad, and I feel privileged to be a fellow-traveler in this exciting field. My deepest gratitude to Graham Farrant who unlocked the doors of primal perception for me—for his afterword and many contributions to this book, and for years of friendship and support in the exploration of new frontiers.

I am grateful to David Chamberlain and Thomas Verny for their helpful criticisms of the manuscript, and for the improvements made by David Cheek and Gayle Peterson to the script of *Inside Experiences*. Many thanks to Terence Dowling for permission to use his guided visualization in Appendix 1.

Ashley Montagu's generous foreword and insightful comments about the text are greatly appreciated, not the least his quip about "psychoclerotics," who will reject the kind of phenomena that I attempt to elucidate! My former editor Barbara Gess, while not present to midwife the book's birth, certainly helped during its gestation—a period of continuing search and discovery. The commitment of Simon & Schuster to such a project was an inspiration.

Michael Noll widened my horizons as we explored the musical corollaries for prenatal development in the production of my audiotape, *Inside Experiences*. I respect his thoroughness in getting the sounds just right.

My long-suffering family survived another book, again created mostly while I breastfed at the computer and at odd hours of the night! My love and thanks to Leo, Julia, and Carsten for their understanding and patience.

Note

Throughout the book I refer to the individual undergoing pre- and perinatal experiences as "he" to avoid confusion with the feminine pronoun, which I reserve for the mother. In keeping with the jargon of the alternative therapies movement, I use the word *primal* as both an adjective and a verb in the more generic sense. Perinatal (from the Greek *peri*, meaning "around, about") refers to the period after birth (medically the first 28 days). The primal period is more inclusive, ranging from conception to language acquisition. The use of the term *regression* refers to age regression—going back to the primal period from conception through infancy. Individuals referred to by a first name include my own clientele, clients of Graham Farrant and other therapists, plus anecdotes from phone calls and letters. Those names have been changed to protect their privacy.

Contents

Foreword

Elizabeth Noble's *Primal Connections* is a remarkable and important book, remarkable because it is as if a scientist had set out to explore a *terra incognita,* and returned to write an account of discoveries incredible as they were exciting, important because the hitherto unknown world thus revealed holds every promise to teach us what we need to understand concerning the personal universe in which we come into being. For what Ms. Noble ably sets out before us are the grounds and reasons for believing that the psychological experiences that we undergo in the womb will influence our behavior for the rest of our lives.

It was in 1642 that Sir Thomas Browne, in *Religio Medici,* wrote, "And surely we are all out of the computation of our age, and every man is some months elder than he bethinks him; for we live, move, and have a being, and are subject to the actions of the elements, and the malice of diseases, in that other world, the truest Microcosm, the womb of our mother." Reading those words in 1802, Samuel Taylor Coleridge remarked in *Miscellanies: Aesthetic and Literary,* "This is a most admirable passage. Yes,—the history of man for the nine months preceding his birth, would, probably, be far more interesting, and contain certain events of greater moment, than all the three-score and ten years that follow it."

Interestingly enough such insights as those of Browne and Coleridge were not again to recur until the twentieth century, principally with the advent of Freud and psychoanalysis. In our own time considerable interest has developed about the psychic life of the organism in the womb; a number of books as well as journals have been devoted to the subject, but Ms. Noble's book is by far the most thorough and extensive, as well as the most challenging.

The field of prenatal influences is a difficult one, and much of its theory is based on speculation, which has often not been subject to the kind of proof that the scientist demands. The reader should not be overworried by this, for speculation is the lifeblood of the scientist, the golden guess, as it were, to the full round of truth. The scientist believes in proof without certainty, while others believe in certainty without proof. But before we can get to proof one must speculate, even fantasize. The trick, of course, is not to fall into the error of mistaking one's speculations or fantasies for facts or certainties. Ms. Noble believes that what she writes is for the most part probable, even though she does at times write as if she were certain. I am glad she does, for if she didn't believe that she was searching for truths in an important and largely unexplored territory, we should not have had this fascinating and admirable book.

—Ashley Montagu

Introduction

I have worked with childbearing families for more than twenty years, learning more about life and love from them than I ever would have expected. After graduating from college in Australia, I worked and traveled in Europe and Asia for almost four years. After my return to Australia I went back to college to study anthropology and philosophy, which, together with part-time work at a maternity teaching hospital, allowed me to link my interests in these three fields. Obstetrics and gynecology were part of my undergraduate training in physical therapy. My anthropology research focused on factors of support and stress in unwed mothers, who in the early 1970s were still relinquishing their babies for adoption; abortion in Australia was illegal then.

While I pursued my studies, I began a private practice specializing in obstetrical and gynecological physical therapy. I offered childbirth preparation classes for expectant couples, as well as treatment for orthopedic problems during pregnancy and postpartum, and gynecological conditions. I spent time in labor and delivery, and began to question many birth practices from philosophical, psychological, and physiological points of view.

In 1973, my husband and I moved to the United States, where this branch of physical therapy was quite undeveloped.

For instance, maternity hospitals didn't have physical therapy departments, in contrast to other English-speaking and European countries. When no hospital in Boston would employ me as an OB-GYN physical therapist, I began work in a rehabilitation hospital. After much searching, I was accepted to teach evening childbirth classes in a suburban Boston hospital. My interest in early pregnancy education, especially prenatal exercise, led to the publication of my first book in 1976, and in 1977 I founded the Obstetrics and Gynecology Section of the American Physical Therapy Association.

I also wanted to create a haven for pregnant and postpartum women. In 1979, partner Linda Gallagher and I started the Maternal and Child Health Center in Cambridge—a private clinic specializing in educational and therapeutic services for expectant and new parents. Within a year of opening the center, I became pregnant, as a result of donor insemination, after five years of infertility. Confidently, I planned for a home birth in Ottawa, where my husband at the time was working, and took maternity leave for the last two months to end the commuting.

The unexpected and distressing events of my birth experience proved to be a turning point in my life. I went into labor three weeks early and then labor "stopped." After eighteen hours of a fully dilated cervix, contractions had not returned and I agreed to enter the hospital. Subsequent events led to a quick case of "cut, yank, and sew." I was furious at the obstetrician whom I had met only minutes before as well as puzzled by the course of my labor, which had stopped *at home*. No one had intervened; painfully, I had to assume the responsibility myself.

Feelings of anger and frustration persisted after that birth. My colleagues in the childbirth field shed no light on the reasons, either. In my own practice, I had reached a point where I was no longer content to treat a patient's symptoms, to provide a quick fix. Rather, I longed to know the reason *why* a client had a certain problem—why at that point in *time* and why in that particular *area* of the body. And of course, for myself, there were many "whys" about my labor. I sensed that there was some meaning to it all, perhaps a chance to heal the past and maybe to reach out and help others. But I felt a wall around me that blocked any enlightenment.

In 1983 I returned to Australia for a lecture tour. One of the participants in my Sydney workshop was a senior physical therapist, who described her recent serious car accident. I was astonished when she stated that she had since undergone psychotherapy that had enabled her to connect that accident to *her birth*. The unresolved frustration from her experience of being born (or, rather, being stuck) was reenacted: her head banging against her mother's pelvis in a long, obstructed labor drove her decades later into a head-on collision. I was incredulous, although her calm tone of complete conviction impressed me deeply.

As a result of this encounter I was curious to meet Dr. Graham Farrant, the psychiatrist who had helped her. Fortunately, I was heading for Melbourne and called to arrange a meeting with him. My subsequent journey into my primal realms during an "intensive" the following year is described in this book. I was able to clear the "wall" I felt around me (it related back to the "wall of fear" around my mother's egg) and identify other issues about my conception and gestation that had blocked my labor. As a result, five years afterward, I successfully experienced both conception and birth, naturally instead of artificially.

Thus, my labor experience was a catalyst for my professional development as well as my personal growth. When the unresolved issues from my primal period were relived, understood, and integrated, I not only healed the trauma of my first birth but several intergenerational issues in my family as well. I continue to become increasingly convinced that the formative period in the uterus holds the key to many subsequent events and experiences—careers and relationships as well as dysfunction and disease.

The Chinese have always considered the period of gestation in calculating a person's age. Nine months is a long time to stay in one place; we leave the uterus with all kinds of uncon-

scious assumptions about ourselves and the world we are entering. Parents and hospital staff agree that every newborn is
different. Some babies enter the world feeling that it is a safe,
welcoming place; others feel that it is dangerous because they
have been hurt—held upside down, forced to breathe with a
tube in their throat, for example. But even earlier there are
definite imprints, also known as *engrams* or *memory matrices*,
that are impressed onto the unconscious mind. Many adults,
especially women, have a feeling that their parents desired the
opposite gender. It is very common for individuals to sense that
the pregnancy was unwanted. These feelings, as we shall see,
go right back to embryonic days and give rise to such "personal
laws" as "females are inferior" and "I am a burden." Thus,
prenatal experiences can form the basis for *life scripts*—limiting
attitudes that hold back a person's true potential.

I empathize with the reader who feels it is far-fetched to
claim that the embryo experiences such feelings and assumptions. I was a skeptic myself until the evidence proved me wrong
and drove me to the research that I share in this book. In the
following chapters I convey some of the convincing data for
the existence of earliest memory, not just of birth but before
—going back to egg and sperm. I outline the development of
this new branch of human understanding, dealing with both
anecdotal material and scientific confirmation, so that readers
can appreciate the broad foundation on which these inner experiences rest. These early memories can be profound; they are
indelibly registered with adrenalin and other hormones released
in deep emotional states.

Making connections with the origins of our attitudes and
"personal laws" is the way the puzzle is pieced together. This
is an essential process to integrate the primal experiences with
the conscious mind and to begin changing old patterns. Connections emerge as an "Aha!" kind of knowing, accompanied
by a satisfying sense of conviction—the revitalization of one's
personal reality. Reliving an obstructed labor, for example, can
relieve a person's anxiety and claustrophobia preventing the
use of elevators, or banish decades of shoulder pain if that body

part had been the cause of the obstruction. Migraine headaches often go away after a person recalls the pressure in the birth canal or a forceps delivery. Relationships may be seen in a new light when one goes back to the first attachment (uterine implantation) with one's mother. Infertility problems may be resolved when a woman gets in touch with the fear of and resistance to her own conception or an unresolved pre- or perinatal loss.

The elevation of fetal memory into higher neural pathways for translation into language is amazing; how is it that he or she can describe pre- and perinatal events, and even repeat conversations verbatim? The mechanism of memory storage and retrieval continues to elude us; it remains a mystery how cellular and out-of-body experiences (when memory is formed while completely absent from body cells), often verifiable, can be recalled. Yet impressive evidence of such memories is accumulating and being confirmed by parents and hospital staff who were present at the time. Current theories and research into memory and brain-mind relationships give increasing credence to memories of pre- and perinatal events.

When connections are made, a person can then *act* with the full consciousness of an adult, rather than unconsciously *act out* patterns laid down as a vulnerable fetus or newborn.

Individuals, of course, unfold in myriad ways, but in my experience with those who choose to take this route, the value of accessing primal memories in relieving confusion, unhappiness, disease, and dysfunction is impressive. Reaching back to one's earliest and deepest feelings is terrifying at first, but it is ultimately liberating. Sometimes nothing less will allow completion of "unfinished business," with its repressed anger or restrained grief. Profound existential issues arise about the continuity of consciousness, with questions such as "Who am I"? "Why am I here?" "Where did I come from?" "Where will I go?" "Did I choose this existence, these parents?" Cultures connect these fundamental biological and spiritual experiences through myths and legends. Symbols representing birth and prenatal states appear in religions, dreams, metaphors—any aspect of human creation—as we journey from womb to tomb.

Feeling the levels of my own fear and pain was a necessary initiation to developing my interest in and understanding of pre- and perinatal psychology. In 1985 I returned to Graham Farrant's clinic to observe and interview his clients for this book, and since that time I have facilitated my own clients' inner journeys. Many case histories are described here, illustrating a wide range of pre- and perinatal experiences. Thus there are three themes woven through this book: 1) my personal journey, 2) an exploration of the phenomena of age regression, and 3) new developments in the exciting field of pre- and perinatal psychology.

Various approaches that enable a person to access these early memories are considered, such as primal therapy, hypnosis, visualization, and bodywork. *Abreaction*—emotional discharges such as shaking and sweating—as well as specific sensations of pressure or pain often occur with bodywork such as deep massage, energy balancing, and breathing techniques. Sometimes a person gains an insight after an inner exploration through a drawing or by writing a poem, rather than by speaking. Completing a personal history questionnaire and genogram (family tree of life events; see Appendix 1) is a fruitful undertaking for the conscious mind. This experience usually motivates a person to search further and deeper.

I have included a guided recall, with cues of taste, touch, sound, and sight, as an initial foray into the unconscious mind's storehouse of emotions and memory of events at birth and during the months before. One partner can read the visualization to the other, or both can participate by listening to the audiotape (see Resources). This is merely an introduction, of course. A skillful and experienced guide who has come to terms with his or her own fear and vulnerability *at the preverbal and prenatal level* can create an environment of safety and support to allow deeper regression in the client.

This book is written for those people who have suffered a lifetime of emotional and/or physical symptoms. Chronic dysfunction or disease, unremitting despite a variety of treatments

with a multitude of providers, strongly suggests prenatal or perinatal causes.

One doesn't have to be in a crisis or have a specific motivating
problem, of course. Rewarding insights into present-day relationships invariably result from journeying back to one's primal
past. This work is important for parents to break patterns
and scripts that often reverberate through generations. Obtain-
ing, or failing to obtain, information from family members
or medical records can arouse a strong desire to discover the
truth.

This book is also directed toward pregnant women and their
partners, because an individual's own experiences of conception, gestation (development in the womb), and birth are far
more influential than any intellectual education about these
events. Expectant parents will become more aware of the per-
sonhood of their own unborn baby as they bring to consciousness
some of their own primal realities.

The months of pregnancy provide an opportunity to begin
the process of healing and resolution. (Ideally, a woman or her
partner tackle their anxiety and conflict concerning any part
of the childbearing cycle *before* conception.) The questionnaire
and guided visualization in the appendices offer a way to begin.
Labor and delivery are powerful rites of passage, and they stir
up primal feelings, some of which may occur only during pregnancy and birth. During pregnancy, deep emotional expression
on the part of the mother may temporarily distress her unborn
baby (he may kick in protest), but that is preferable to chronic
ambivalence, resentment, or even terror about the pregnancy
or impending birth. Short periods of strong feelings that bring
integration of painful memories are part of the stress and relaxation cycles that form the context of learning.

Certainly for women who have a history of complications in
pregnancy or birth, or who are currently experiencing a problem
such as high blood pressure or preterm labor, connecting to the
origin of the symptom may reduce the need for medication or
even alleviate the condition. Hypnosis, gentle bioenergetics,
or visualizations are sometimes the only way to resolve a high-

risk medical situation, particularly when pharmacological treatment is ineffective.

Parents will find that this book affirms their impulses to bond prenatally with their unborn and newborn babies—to sing, talk, touch. Understanding that the unborn baby is aware and sentient means we have to react to him with much more consideration and respect during pregnancy. The challenge is to use what is known about human potential to broaden prenatal education, and to change birth and postpartum practices that poorly accommodate the baby's sensitivities. Parents who tune in to their unborn baby learn to trust their instincts. This helps them find the courage they need to reject irrational and inhumane practices during the childbearing experience.

TOWARD A KINDER, GENTLER WORLD

Accessing primal experiences in a multitude of ways can ameliorate confusion, unhappiness, disease, and dysfunction in daily life. Getting in touch with our deepest feelings facilitates the completion of unfinished business, which in turn frees us to live more spontaneously and creatively.

In my opinion, such personal journeys can pave the way for social transformation. In a society where everyone blames someone else (parents, teachers, doctors) and litigation is epidemic, the time has come for each person to own his or her own truths, to take responsibility for his or her individual reality. Chilton Pearce warns that "the destruction of technological man will take place no faster through pollution or the bomb, or any kind of weaponry, than through the collapse of the child." And the child begins with sperm and egg.

Pain, hurt, and feelings of intense vulnerability are part of most people's primal journeys. Few of us were consciously and desirously conceived in love and harmony, enjoyed a blissful gestation in a mother free of tension and anxiety, were birthed without medication and anesthesia, and emerged spontaneously into gentle welcoming hands. Fewer of us enjoyed breastfeeding on demand and constant contact with our mother's body after birth. Life in the world was a rude awakening compared to life in the womb; continuity was lacking and our security was threatened. It is imperative that we heal these experiences before we unwittingly repeat them with our children.

In addition, the increasing medicalization of birth has led to escalating obstetric interventions (more than one-fourth of all births in the U.S. are by Cesarean delivery), which compounds the family dynamics. Over a hundred years ago the German philosopher Immanuel Kant wrote of the "cry of wrath at the catastrophe of birth." He would turn in his grave to see how today, in the words of psychiatrist R. D. Laing, "the whole birth process is shredded to pieces by technological intervention . . . a most remarkable feature of our time." We have an urgent double duty: to maximize the child's human potential in utero and to protect him from external assaults by the health care system, however well intentioned.

I believe that when *real* change occurs in how babies are brought into the world, and in the consciousness with which they are received, the levels of addiction, violence, and crime in society will be reduced. The fetal drama that plays behind the curtain within us all also plays on a wider scale, within groups and nations. Personal transformation, then, can have political effects; as psychohistorian Lloyd deMause wrote, "psychological maturation is a historical achievement." It's a matter of starting at the very beginning.

The Renaissance of Prenatal Psychology

The child grows daily more when in the body of its mother than when it is outside of the body, and this teaches us.
— LEONARDO DA VINCI

Imagine that you and I were to spend nine months together in a small enclosed space. At the end of this time you would have many opinions and assumptions about yourself and me. Likewise, each of us leaves the womb with profound impressions that influence the rest of our life.

The frontiers of human experience are expanding all the time. Just as we are hearing more about near-death experiences—the other end of the spectrum—the time of birth and just before is gaining attention in books and the media. But I am amazed at the depth and extent of writing on pre- and perinatal psychology from earlier decades as well. I mention these books with enthusiasm because so few therapists in this field, let alone consumers, realize what they have missed!

The classic work on pre- and perinatal experiences, *The Trauma of Birth*, was written by Otto Rank and was first published in Germany in 1923. Other Europeans followed in the 1940s and 1950s with, for example, Nandor Fodor's *The Search for the Beloved* and Francis Mott's *The Nature of the Self*, as well as *The Universal Design of Birth*, M. L. Peerbolte's *Prenatal Dynamics*, R. D. Laing's *The Facts of Life*, and Frank Lake's *Clinical Theology* and *Tight Corners in Pastoral Counseling*. In the United States, Stan Grof's *Realms of the Human Unconscious* and Lloyd deMause's *Foundations of Psychohistory* carried on this exploration of the deepest biological layer of the unconscious. *Prenatal Influences* by Ashley Montagu, *The Secret Life of the Unborn Child* by Thomas Verny, and *Babies Remember Birth* by David Chamberlain further continued the concept of fetal awareness.

The movie, *Look Who's Talking*, with the ongoing commentary from the unborn baby, was as factual as it was playful, and introduced the prenatal world of emotions and assumptions to a very broad audience. *Aliens* and the two *Terminator* films powerfully depict prenatal symbols and were very successful at the box office.

Researchers today are looking at birth memories from two perspectives: experiences relived by adults in hypnosis and regressive therapies; and scientific studies of the activities of the unborn and newborn child. David Chamberlain has documented parallel recall of birth experiences through hypnosis in mother-child dyads. Gamete cell functions are being studied in the laboratory by infertility researchers while scientists explore the structure of information substances in the nervous system. We also now know that the function of cells is affected by the emotions, which in turn impacts on the hormonal and immune systems. These new sciences—known as psychoneuroendocrinology and psychoneuroimmunology, respectively—are changing the way we view the relationship between mind/brain and body.

The integration of science and psychotherapy is thus expanding the dimensions of human experience, and an evermore fascinating body of knowledge is emerging. The human potential movement provides a context for this heightened appreciation of the indivisible human—the unity of body, mind, and spirit.

PRE- AND PERINATAL METAPHORS

Birth metaphors abound in our daily language. For example, headaches may be described as feeling an "intense pressure" or "waves of tension that come and go." Other metaphors that recall labor are "I felt crushed," "my world is falling in on me," "I have no room to maneuver," "no room to turn," "I feel stifled . . . or smothered," "I'm getting pressure from all sides . . . or all directions." Time and space images such as "I'm in a pinch" or a "tight squeeze," "I'm waiting for a breakthrough," "I feel stuck," and "there's never enough time," "I'm not in a good space right now," "I can't make it alone," "I can't get through it," "There's no way out," "I've got to get out of here," "Don't rush me," "I'm not ready" and "I'm getting in over my head" are also metaphors recalling birth. "No one is here for me," "I took a turn for the worse," "It made a world of difference," and especially "Help me out" relate to birth experiences, too.

Some people say that they have a hard time "getting their head into that space"; others feel they are just "banging their head against a brick wall." Statements like "I can't go on" or "I can't seem to get started" may also compare to labor or birth. Some individuals "put feelers out" while others "dive fearlessly" into things, once they have "found an opening." A person anxious about public speaking may feel "I shall never get to the end of this passage alive."

A common intrauterine metaphor is "hanging in" there, or being "the center of their world" or feeling that "there's nobody there for me." People who say they shouldn't "rock the boat" or "make waves," or that they'll "never be good enough," are describing uterine life. "I could sink into the earth" and "I feel so small I could shrink out of sight," also "sucking up" to people, being "sucked into things" refer to womb existence.

Conception images may be expressed in phrases like "I need to swallow everything whole to take it in," "I can't seem to get into this," "I felt like a little black dot surrounded by millions of people," "My head feels like it is going to explode," "I'm afraid to take the plunge," and "My head is splitting." Describing oneself as a "ball of fear" may relate to the egg or cell mass (blastocyst) anxiety after conception. "I'm just spinning around . . . or spinning my wheels" may refer to the bundle of cells before implantation. "I'm buried with work" suggests implantation, and feeling like a "sponge" is a placental image. Individuals who presented in the birth canal with the lower part of their body (breech) may use expressions such as "I'm backing out of . . ." "I keep putting my foot in my mouth," or "I jump into things feet first." Face presentations at birth may have difficulty "facing up to things" or often say, "Let's face it."

Alternatively, the latter may have to do with a mother's rejecting facial expression after birth. "You're on your own now" is a comment that can bring back early memories of asphyxia or cord-cutting. "What a treat—I don't even know I've been born" indicates that something so good has happened that the trauma of birth can be set aside.

Images and labels are symbols, giving clues to the nature and timing of pre- or perinatal experiences, and they describe actual symptoms. These metaphors may sound amusing to some people, but as hidden persuaders they can perpetuate behavior patterns in later life. Symbols are more than words, and through them a wide range of pre- and perinatal events can be discerned in dreams and myths as well.

THE AMAZING UNBORN

In 1972, William Liley, the New Zealand pioneer of prenatal blood transfusions for blood group incompatibility, expressed his admiration for the "splendidly functioning" perceptions, survival mechanisms, and skills that the unborn develops since conception. Structure and function develop together; it is because of their specialized functions that all the integrated parts unfold with the appropriate design.

Rather than a "witless tadpole with a mind like a cleanly-washed slate," the baby guarantees the success of the pregnancy through hormonal and other physiological changes he initiates, Liley noted. Furthermore, the baby determines the duration of the pregnancy, and decides which way he will lie in pregnancy and present during labor. From about the twelfth week, the baby controls the amount of amniotic fluid by swallowing it. (Nutrients are present in the fluid and contribute to weight gain.) By fourteen weeks, taste buds in his tongue have completed their development.

Canadian psychiatrist Thomas Verny wrote in *The Secret Life of the Unborn Child* that from the sixth month of conception the fetus is sufficiently developed neurologically, with circuits linking the cortex of the brain, to receive, process, and encode information. This is obvious when these babies are born prematurely: they see, feel, hear, and are mentally alert. But this evidence is often denied those of the same gestational age who are still in the uterus.

Those who have observed obstetric ultrasound are aware of the responses of the embryo (the stage of development between the second and eighth weeks) and the fetus (the term for the unborn baby after eight weeks). The embryo will move away from a needle penetrating his uterine world and is often disturbed by douches or swabbing of the vagina for medical procedures. And boys have erections in the uterus! Every parent who looks into the eyes of their newborn knows intuitively that here is an individual with a distinct personality, and mothers of twins often perceive differences between their babies before birth.

THE AMAZING NEWBORN

The baby who suckles, grimaces, grasps, cries, and gazes with wide-open eyes did not suddenly become that way at the moment of birth. He began to learn in the womb. For instance, newborns can select their mother's breast pads from others by their already developed keen sense of smell. Newborns clearly remember music, stories, and songs to which they were exposed in the uterus. Verified memories relating to events experienced in prenatal life, such as concerts, carnivals, train whistles, and explosions, can be found in the literature. In fact, as Chamberlain has pointed out, the abilities of the unborn and newborn seem to expand with the improvements in studying them!

Infants are capable of understanding and responding to language before they can speak (as when an adult learns a foreign language, comprehension comes before speech) and studies show that learning definitely occurs in the uterus. Anthony DeCasper, a psychologist at the University of North Carolina, conducted experiments with women who read three stories to their unborn babies during the last six weeks of pregnancy. After birth, thirteen of the sixteen babies who were tested showed a preference for the familiar story, in contrast to one they had never heard. (The babies were able to switch tapes by changing their sucking rhythm.) Likewise with music.

Thus, babies are able to shape their world, discriminate, recall events, use body language, and learn more in the first year of life than in any subsequent year, all without lessons!

RESISTANCE TO THE EVIDENCE OF PRENATAL AWARENESS

The philosopher Bertrand Russell once was told by a fisherman that fish have no sense or sensation, but how the fisherman knew that the fisherman could not say! So too about babies. Gross ignorance about the sentience and inherent abilities of unborn and newborn babies prevails. Many people still believe that "babies don't think or feel," or that "smiles result from intestinal gas." Yet research has exposed the secret life of plants and their empathetic relationships to humans. Why would a baby in the uterus be less sentient than a flower in a pot?

French obstetrician Frederick LeBoyer gained international fame in the early 1970s for his book *Birth Without Violence*, which led to heightened appreciation for the sensitivities of the newborn. Yet many physicians, neurologists, and research physiologists still insist that because the myelin nerve sheaths are not complete at birth, babies do not feel pain; manifestations of pain have been passed off as reflexes. While I am an advocate for drugless birth, I find it an interesting bias that only maternal pain relief has been considered in birth and for postpartum "after pains." Yet birth and the days following are very often painful and traumatic for the baby. Anyone who accidentally pricks a baby with a diaper pin knows that it hurts him! Even today in the United States, minor and even major surgery is still performed on newborns without anesthesia (circumcision is only one example). Babies who were circumcised will often scream in terror for a long time afterward when their diapers are removed; they still remember the pain.

Why has it taken so long to develop this awareness of unborn and newborn children? Why do we resist the concept of prenatal consciousness? Outmoded theories of memory, taboos around birth, and prejudice against women and infants play a large role. Frequently, there are deep guilt feelings associated with being born, both feeling and causing pain, and with giving birth. Francis Mott suggested that feelings of the womb can also be incestuous and that denial is the barrier that insulates against such emotions.

Birth arouses our existential anxiety about the meaning of life. Belief in the consciousness of the unborn often raises fears in people about what may be harbored in their own buried primal memories. One result of gaining this knowledge and insight is that we regret our prior ignorance. "If only . . ." is a natural reaction, although not a constructive one. Some mothers feel guilty about their emotions and actions during pregnancy and birth. This is often part of a generational pattern, which when understood and explored can provide valuable insights into family history. Guilt, which arises from continued identification with past mistakes, can be transformed into healing by understanding life's lessons or appreciating that an experience is universal rather than just personal.

Some feminists worry that the mounting evidence confirming the "humanness" of the fetus or embryo will strengthen opposition to abortion. Thomas Verny, who also founded the Pre and Perinatal Psychology Association of North America, reassured women in a 1989 issue of *Omni* magazine, that although pre- and perinatal psychology obviously focuses on reproductive issues, it does *not* represent any political movement to take away a woman's right to choose. I would add that awareness of prenatal consciousness makes us realize how important it is that babies are planned and welcomed. Studies have confirmed that individuals born to mothers whose requests for abortion were denied grow up to lead unhappy lives. Such research strengthens the pro-choice position. A slogan of the pro-lifers, "The most dangerous place to grow in America is in a mother's womb," ironically proves the same point.

Male bias in Western anthroplogy and medicine has seriously limited our understanding of mothers and babies. Participation by fathers at delivery in Western culture is relatively recent, and the male obstetrician has usurped the role of the midwife only in the last hundred years. In our technological society, reproduction is becoming less of a rite of passage that affirms and values the experience of the individuals involved. Instead, as described by anthropologist Robbie Davis-Floyd, medicalized rituals have evolved that depersonalize all members of the family unit. Davis-Floyd has exposed the American way of birth as primarily an initiation into technological society.

SPONTANEOUS RECALL OF PRE-
AND PERINATAL EVENTS
BY CHILDREN

I remember many years ago an obstetrician's surprise when a mother came with her three-year-old child and the little girl remarked, "Crowning . . . crowning," which were the exact words he had spoken as her head emerged. Although such experiences are quite common, adults tend to laugh them off instead of taking the opportunity to affirm and explore this phenomenon. When birth recall is met with disbelief, further spontaneous recall by the child is shut down and the memories slip into the unconscious.

Children have recalled verifiable details such as the color of the doctor's shoes and details of the delivery room or the type of wallpaper and furniture in a home birth. Other memories, which are also verifiable, include individuals present or absent, especially fathers, as well as remarks made.

For over a decade now, pregnant women in my classes have been informed about this natural ability of very young children and are encouraged to ask for more details via open-ended questions. Many mothers of young children have reported, with great excitement, that there was indeed accurate recall. One child, delivered by instruments after a second-stage arrest, told her mother "I didn't want to come out. I didn't feel ready, so I turned and put my arms like this," demonstrating on the floor the exact position of her body when labor failed to progress.

New York psychiatrist Rima Laibow related how her young son was sitting in the bath one day and asked why at his birth he saw only "half-faces," referring to the surgical masks at his Cesarean delivery. He also imitated the sound of the suction equipment.

A bath may facilitate intrauterine memories. My daughter Julia loved to go underwater to remember her birth. Even as late as the age of eight, I would ask her questions like "Which shoulder came out first?" "Which breast did you nurse at first?"

and "When you were in my belly was the cord already cut or not?" She was always right. Also, at the age of four, she described her artificial insemination conception, in terms that were quite explicit and unlike any adult description.

As this exciting field develops, we must be careful to avoid stereotypes concerning birth trauma. For example, beliefs that menopausal babies are judgmental, that Cesareans can't complete a task without outside help, or that forceps babies have to be dragged through life. Not all Cesareans insist on quick solutions, and not all people born vaginally push ahead! An individual born vaginally may have the same personal law or life script as one born by Cesarean. The varieties of pre- and perinatal experiences are infinite. Each person's reality is unique, and a similar event can also have different ramifications in different people.

One day, when Julia was about five, I asked her how she was born—whether she was pushed or pulled out. She said "pulled."

I asked by whom.

"The doctor," she replied, "a man." Next, she demonstrated with her hands on her head exactly where the forceps were placed, "with something on my head."

To test her, I put my hands front and back instead and said, "Wasn't it like this?"

"No," she said, "like this," putting her hands correctly at the sides of her temples again.

"How did that feel?" I continued.

"Tight," replied Julia.

"Did it hurt?" I asked.

"No, it was just tight."

She loves to wear hats and headbands, so for her the experience apparently did not leave a negative imprint. I always try to be mindful of the fact that it was my ego that was bruised rather than her head, and thus avoid projecting my reality on to her.

NEW FRONTIERS IN PSYCHOLOGY

Most readers are familiar with Freud's separation of the unconscious and conscious parts of the mind, and his theory that unconscious material nevertheless influences our behavior and relationships. Prior to Freud, Joseph Breuer stressed the fundamental fact that symptoms of hysterical patients depend on impressive but forgotten scenes in their lives. A forgotten psychic injury or guilt materializes in a chronic physical complaint or a physical injury, which then gives rise to a psychological problem. Freud followed this physiological concept with a psychological one—his "doctrine of defence" (sic), which causes the repression of trauma. The origin of anxiety is blocked from consciousness and results in neurosis, or disconnection from the feelings that were experienced during an early trauma. This split sets up a pattern for later reactions to be displaced in the same way. Freud's investigations into both the repressed content and the repressing forces (conscience, guilt feelings, ideals) led to his classification of the id, ego, and superego.

Freud perceived that some of his patients seemed to regress to periods of early development, and would report dreams or feelings of floating in water, or of being in chests and boxes, or would describe being pressed through narrow spaces. He arrived at the idea of birth anxiety at a dinner party where interns were joking about a midwife who failed her examination because she explained the significance of meconium in the amniotic fluid as "the child is frightened." Freud silently took her side, suspecting that "the poor unsophisticated woman's unerring perception had revealed a very important connection."

While Freud wrote that birth anxiety is the prototype for all other anxiety, and that trauma will cause regression to earlier traumas, he left it to his followers to develop theories about prenatal consciousness. Otto Rank concluded that anxiety at birth forms the basis of every anxiety or fear, so "*every pleasure has as its final aim the re-establishment of the intrauterine primal pleasure*" (italics his). Birth, then, is a "violent adventure that uproots our prenatal world," according to Nandor Fodor. The birth of a baby is the death of a fetus, as the German writer Goethe said, a "dying and coming into being." Likewise, near-death experiences have much in common with birth (such as traveling through tunnels and coming into the light).

The Russian physiologist Ivan Pavlov agreed that anxiety experienced at birth retains its influence. He established that the tolerance of the newborn organism to stress in any given stage of infancy is diminished by previous painful stress. There is a tendency to "equate any hurt with total annihilation," as we will see in Chapter 4 with regard to myths and legends. Early hurts from the outside tend to be assimilated into primary fears. Subsequent life transitions such as weaning, leaving home, finishing school, or getting married may provoke equivalent anxiety and resistance. Rank and Fodor both considered negative experiences during the intrauterine stage, including fear of extinction from abortion attempts, the "invading father" during intercourse, or a mother's hostility, as anxieties that "can be woven into a perinatal drama."

Ashley Montagu points out that arousal of the respiratory and cardiovascular systems of the infant at birth organizes patterns of anxiety responses in later life. Gestalt therapist Fritz Perls defined anxiety as the "experience of breathing difficulty during any blocked excitement." Psychologist Rollo May explained it as "a state of human being in the struggle against anything that would destroy his being." Symptoms include nausea, palpitation, diarrhea, frequency of urination, trembling, cold sweats, tightness in head or chest, and genital tension. Anxiety is general and more elusive than fear. Fear is specific, an emotional reaction to a threat to security, and may be an actual phobia. Any fear that we cannot rationalize can lead to panic.

Michel Odent refers to a primal adaptive system that develops and matures during the period from conception through to the end of infancy. Events during this time influence the programs in our biological computers, the "thermostat" for our hormonal levels. For example, separation of a newborn baby from his mother can cause a high secretion of the stress hormone cortisol, which will actually reduce the size of the thymus and suppress the immune system. Feelings are absorbed from the mother, and sometimes the father; the unborn child cannot distinguish between feelings directed toward him and feelings directed toward others. He has no skills to deflect, contain, modify, or release the encompassing emotions. A shock or acute condition sets in motion a different dynamic from a chronic situation, which often produces an attitude of resignation.

During the primal period (conception to about age three), we are completely vulnerable and helpless in the presence of conflicting realities and the internal confusion that results. We deal with physical and emotional trauma by repression—splitting off a part of the self. The core negative experiences are hidden in a deep place and then forgotten.

We live our lives *as if* those core experiences didn't exist. This state of denial means we cannot be entirely real; some of our most profound aspects of personal reality are blocked. The pain resulting from a denied need in early life becomes repressed by various defense mechanisms, including transfer of the traumatic experience into areas of the body. The tension builds until it manifests itself in dysfunction or disease, years or even decades later. At this point we need to make deeper sense of the early frustrating or disappointing experiences.

Robin K. Murray, at the National Institute of Mental Health, reported in 1991 that almost half of schizophrenics had a history of birth complications. Psychiatrists Stanislav Grof and Graham Farrant have both compiled impressive clinical evidence of memories that go back to even *before* conception. Just as psychological exploration that does not go back to birth thus ignores a major event, deeper insights can be gained when individuals regress to the separate existences of sperm and egg, and the quality of their union during fertilization.

For over twenty years, Graham has used his own adaptation of primal therapy to access preverbal and prenatal experiences. He extended the use of the term *primal* back to implantation, fertilization, and even before—coining the term "cellular consciousness" for the memories of individual gametes (egg and sperm). Graham was reluctant to discuss his early insights into sperm and egg behavior for fear of ridicule by his staff and patients. However, as Grof points out, reports of subjects who have experienced episodes of embryonal existence, conception, and gamete consciousness abound with accurate details about the anatomical, physiological, and biochemical processes involved.

The late Frank Lake, a psychiatrist and pastoral counselor in Nottingham, England, described in detail the emotional connection flowing between mother and baby via the umbilical cord. He placed the mother's emotions on a continuum from positive to negative. From conception onward, suggested Lake, the unborn baby has a "shopping list and hopes for [a] 'well-stocked' maternal shop." In the best circumstances the fetus experiences oceanic bliss and a sense of inherent goodness. However, when the unborn baby's needs for adequate growth and development are not met, the baby becomes confused about his reality and a split occurs. Instead of a sense of connection, of unity and wholeness, a duality results. This split happens at any point along the continuum of life—egg and sperm, fertilized egg (blastocyst) and implantation, fetus and birth, newborn and the breast. Lake emphasized the period of gestation. If the fetus feels that maternal emotion or "umbilical affect" (that is, the emotions funneled to the baby) is negative, he feels unrecognized and insignificant. Sometimes a situation develops wherein the baby feels that if he gives up his energy and vitality he will receive something in exchange. These babies feel they have had their energy and life drained out of them and tend to feel drained again under stress in later life. Lake stated that this pattern of "giving in order to get" remains throughout life.

Liley pointed out that babies with severe growth retardation "make it hard to believe that every foetus [sic] lives in a metabolic Nirvana . . . with an obliging mother and faithful placenta supplying the baby's every need."

In 1970, Arthur Janov published his landmark work, The Primal Scream, which initiated the primal therapy movement. In a 1983 book, Imprints: The Lifelong Effects of the Birth Experience, Janov outlined in more detail how physical and emotional problems are connected to birth. Both pain and its response are engraved into the nervous system; they become unified so that under later stress the original response pattern, consisting of the same quality of emotion and the same defense mechanisms, is automatically triggered. Rather than eliminating or conquering the feelings that constitute our lives, the journey is to rediscover those feelings, staying with the fear, the frustration, the inadequacy, as deeply and completely as possible in order to let those feelings take us back to the primal trauma.

Fear, which I believe is the basis of all human emotions, keeps us disconnected from feeling the rage and frustration of formative early experiences. Thus it is fear we need to overcome in order to understand the truth of our own reality, whether it was being unwanted, being the wrong gender, having survived abortion attempts, or losing a twin. When we understand that emotional blocks correspond with physical symptoms, mobilizing this blocked energy into a flow of dynamic experiences brings healing on many levels.

The unborn baby experiences his mother's emotions whether she is anxious, angry, relaxed, joyful, sick, or feeling the effects of drugs or alcohol. Marvin Colter wrote:

The fetus is a "captive audience" beyond the dreams of the most fanatic brainwasher. Never again in the long life of the person will his mind and his body be more vulnerable. For it is truly in the womb, where impinging stimuli and cellular growth are inextricably and inescapably mixed, where self-defense is unthinkable, that those life experiences yet to come are indeed fore-ordained, where the personality receives the primary, the basic, the core-level engrams that will shape the content of the person's life, perhaps unalterably. Perhaps it is here, in the womb, bathed in the fluid distillate of parental anxieties, hopes, ambivalence and fears, that the basic shape of the personality is laid down.

Years earlier, Lester Sontag observed:

To all intents and purposes a neurotic infant when he is born is the result of an unsatisfactory foetal [sic] environment. In this instance he has not had to wait until childhood for a bad home situation or other cause to make him neurotic. It has been done for him before he has even seen the light of day.

As we will see later, information substances flow through the body to link memory and learning, and certain states are dependent upon emotions and other responses to the environment for their physiological qualities. The receptors in the unborn baby are affected by hormones or chemicals produced by the nervous and immune systems. The placenta functions like a sieve, not a filter; thus mothers who consume liquor in pregnancy may have babies with fetal alcohol syndrome, and mothers who smoke will send their babies into respiratory distress, observed with ultrasound, even if they just *think* about reaching for a cigarette.

In anticipation of maternal guilt, let me reassure women with such feelings that the mother's emotions are not the whole picture. Genes are seen to play an increasing role in determining human temperament and health. Twin research has shown that two babies in the same uterine environment have very different personalities. However, genetic manipulation is not available for the average person; on the other hand, education, self-awareness, and communication with the unborn child are. Hence my commitment to disseminating information about pre- and perinatal psychology.

Pre- and perinatal psychology has much to offer conventional psychiatrists and psychologists, who traditionally engage in verbal exchanges with clients sitting upright in a chair and making eye contact. The significant primal material is rarely tapped because, by definition, it is preverbal and inaccessible through ordinary conversation. However, memories from birth and before often emerge within professional interactions when lying down, closure of eyes, and touch are integral to the treatment. Expression of repressed emotions may occur spontaneously during physical therapy, massage, and other bodywork, depending on the degree of empathy and safety experienced by the client. Hypnosis and visualization offer great possibilities for psychologists who do not engage in bodywork.

Psychotherapists are not usually trained or may not even be permitted to use physical contact, while physical bodyworkers are usually not prepared or educated to provide emotional support in guiding the client's regression. This is a dilemma in our society, which perceives the mind and body as separate and where medicial specialization is highly developed.

UNITING OBSTETRICS WITH PRE- AND PERINATAL PSYCHOLOGY

The mind-body dichotomy is most striking in the field of obstetrics and gynecology, one of the most conservative branches of medicine. I came to accept and endorse Graham's belief that unresolved personal issues surrounding pregnancy and birth lead many, if not most, maternity-care providers into their chosen field. It had always struck me as ironic that the professionals who have the most knowledge about labor and birth are the ones who invariably have the most complications with their own experiences. "We teach what we need to learn" is an appropriate saying. However, with pregnancy and birth, the situation is complex because the practitioners' unconscious need for their own healing has contributed to their increasing interventions in the birth process. Many obstetricians and midwives today were victims of complicated pregnancies and traumatic births, so they (unconsciously and with the best of intentions) chose a field where they can rescue babies from similar trauma. However, the interventions they use (including induction of labor, narcotics, anesthesia, instrumental deliveries, Cesarean section, and heroic measures in neonatal intensive care units) are themselves traumatic and create a reservoir of primal pain and anger for the unborn child. Expectant parents must be aware that pregnancy, labor, and delivery often trigger unconscious pain for nurses, midwives, and doctors who attend them, which may result in a lack of support or, worse, unnecessary procedures. It is difficult for a nurse or doctor who is repressing personal fears of birth or other primal anxieties to affirm rather than direct a laboring woman. As a result, their common reaction is busywork, rescue with drugs, or bossy direction, such as shouting at the mother to push.

Just when birth has never been so medicalized as well as regulated by state legislation, insurance companies, and other bureaucratic systems, the timely rebirth of prenatal and perinatal psychology is urging us to consider as deeply and widely as possible the effects of such interventions on the babies who will inherit our world.

CHAPTER TWO

The Catalyst for My Inner Journey

Every act of birth requires the courage to let go of something, to let go of the breath, to let go of the lap, to let go of the hand, to let go eventually of all certainties and to rely on one's own power to be aware and to respond to that with one's creativity. To be creative is to consider the whole process of life as a process of birth and not to take any stage as the final stage.

—ERICH FROMM

I was born quickly and easily at home, and I never felt that I suffered any trauma. In later years I was grateful that my mother had neither medication nor anesthesia. Our family belief was that birth is uncomplicated, and I expected that my births would be, too. I didn't know then that, while there may have been no skeletons in the birth closet, there were plenty in the uterus!

Being pregnant was the most expansive and blissful feeling I could ever imagine. Growing new life brought me in touch with the creative power of the universe. I felt deeply integrated and content. I luxuriated in a whole-body massage on Mondays and a foot massage on Fridays. My husband Geoff would come home each day for lunch. I took maternity leave for the last two months from my practice in Cambridge, and from the commute to Ottawa, savoring the time I had for physical exercise, listening to music, communicating with the baby inside me, and napping.

We had found a family practitioner in Ottawa who attended births at home, which was for me the only place to feel safe. The pregnancy progressed normally and I was in robust health. A few pessimists thought that at age thirty-six, I should have amniocentesis, but intuitively I felt sure that our baby was just fine, and a girl. She was conceived laboriously with donor insemination, and I was not about to question her existence by undergoing prenatal tests to examine her chromosomes.

My labor began at thirty-seven weeks, several hours after my husband had left for an extended business trip to the United States. I awoke in the middle of a Sunday night and found I was bleeding. The sight of bright red blood filled me with terror.* I made my way to the phone and tried to contact my husband. The operator informed me that the business colleague he was visiting in St. Louis had an unlisted number. Trembling, I sobbed to the operator that I was "hemorrhaging in a foreign country" and begged her to put me through or ask them to call me back. In due course a call came from Geoff, and I asked him to come back as soon as possible. I was afraid that the placenta might be separating prematurely, which would mean a Cesarean. There was nothing he could do at 3 A.M. but wait for the first flight out in the morning.

I swallowed a couple of glasses of white wine to prevent the onset of contractions and dozed fitfully. At about seven in the morning Geoff called from Chicago with the bad news that all flights had been delayed by snowstorms. Furthermore, the Ottawa airport was closed that morning for the first U.S. presidential visit to that city.

Fortunately, the bleeding seemed to stop. I hoped that it was just a separation of a marginal sinus of the placenta (a little piece that grows separately at the edge). At 9 A.M. sharp, I phoned my general practitioner, who said he might be able to schedule an ultrasound that week. "That week," I exclaimed in distress and disbelief, "in Boston you can get an ultrasound immediately!"

Time dragged on until around lunchtime, when I heard Geoff turn the key in the door. As I walked to meet him, my membranes burst and out shot a big clot landing in front of us on the rug. I put it in a jar and decided to go to the clinic for the

* I was later to learn the primal reason for this reaction, which led me into physical therapy and childbirth education, rather than medicine or midwifery, where I would have to deal with loss of blood.

doctor's opinion. My first contraction began as we drove. The doctor was satisfied that the clot was "old and organized," and sent us home to rest. Exhausted as we both were, sleep was impossible with intermittent contractions now underway.

I was extremely reluctant to give birth early. I loved being pregnant and wasn't ready to end that experience. Our doctor kept reminding us that the longer I could keep her inside, the more mature her lungs would be. I was also concerned about whether I could give birth at home three weeks before the due date—usually an indication for transfer to the hospital.

With occasional sips of wine and rest, the contractions remained intermittent and two more days passed. We checked my pulse and temperature for signs of infection, in view of the ruptured membranes. The doctor visited each day, and around lunchtime on Wednesday he checked my cervix for the first time. "One centimeter?" I inquired despondently. "Yep," he said. "That's all." However, an hour or so after he left the contractions became much stronger. I soon had to stand up against the wall, rocking and wailing, yielding to the birth energy like a tree in a storm. I couldn't stand in a warm shower, as I had recommended to others for years, because the hot water system in the apartment building had failed. The elevator was also out of order and we lived on the nineteenth floor!

The period until full dilation was intense, lasting about four hours. Visualizing a rising golden sun helped my cervix to open, despite its being "unripe" (in contrast with a cervix at term, which has been softened by hormones for a quicker, easier dilation).

As I was standing and vocalizing almost entirely throughout the first stage of my labor, the urge to push developed soon after the final dilating contractions. It was about 5:30 P.M. when I felt this sudden change. The energy was so strong, so linear, so downward that I felt pulled toward the floor. I envisaged the baby arriving in seconds on the cold bathroom tiles. I yelled to Geoff to call the doctor. He wanted to argue the point as to whether I was *really* ready to push . . . was I sure? Perhaps I was making a premature request for the doctor?

I became frozen with rage and fear—so powerful that the expulsive contractions that would have brought my baby in minutes into the world came to a wrenching halt. I was furious at not being believed, at having to argue my inner knowing. I was irate at having to get my head together to argue with my husband that birth was imminent instead of surrendering to my body and the process of birth. I felt a complete shift in gear as this duality developed in my awareness. I was now outside the process; "it" had stopped. There is another alternative to fight or flight—it is *fright*, and that was my block.

Effective contractions never returned. By the time I had persuaded Geoff to call and the doctor had arrived, I felt as if I had never been in labor. It was the dinner hour, but I wasn't hungry and the doctor didn't want any food, either. I felt uncomfortably inadequate as a hostess; and I knew he felt detained to watch the proverbial pot that never boils.

I experienced very occasional contractions during which it felt right to be on my hands and knees. Optimistically, I made sure that hot compresses were ready for my perineum when the baby's head came down. After waiting a couple of hours, the doctor asked if he could leave, since he was scheduled to give a lecture at his clinic.

On my insistence, he most reluctantly canceled the lecture. I had been fully dilated already for so long and surely the baby would come soon. We had no other friends or colleagues for support in Ottawa and I did not want him to leave. I knew I would remember my labor and birth until my deathbed, long after he would forget the lecture on hypoglycemia that he never gave.

As the evening dragged on, we tried all kinds of home remedies to get my motor running again—an enema, blue cohosh tea, and reflexology (stimulation of key areas on the feet). Hours passed, but there was only an occasional flutter, never a real contraction. My vital signs and the baby's remained fine. There was no sense of panic; for me it was like being out in the

Australian bush with a broken-down car; nothing to do but
wait.

Then another crisis arose: I couldn't urinate. I had tried to
ignore this problem for the first few attempts, but hearing the
two men get up periodically to pee with the toilet door ajar
mocked my frustration. The more I tried to pee, the more I
felt I couldn't, not even with running water.

After boiling a large rubber tube on our kitchen stove,
the doctor catheterized my bladder, which by now was bulging
over my pubic bone. It was an agonizing invasion, but a relief
to let go of the pressure. A few hours later, however, my
bladder was painfully bursting again. But this time my urethra
went into such spasm it was not possible for the doctor to
insert the catheter despite lubrication and all our relaxation techniques. I simply wouldn't let it in. He went to his
clinic and found a much smaller catheter that I could
accommodate. Why had he not brought that size the first time?
I cursed.

Before dawn the doctor decided he wanted to go home and
sleep. He called in a midwife whom I had never met. She bedded
down on our living room sofa to await some action.

By breakfast time on Thursday I really felt I had never started
labor, except that with the amniotic fluid gone my belly was
the most remarkable sight. It was as if a wet cloth had been
placed over the baby, making all her body contours visible.
The doctor returned and wanted to consult an obstetrician. I
called an old friend and colleague (now my husband), Leo
Sorger, in Boston, to whom the doctor reported that my membranes had been ruptured for over three days and that I had
been fully dilated for fifteen hours without further progress. The
obstetrician's advice was to get the baby out by noon to avoid
infection. My doctor reassured me about his back-up specialist:
an Asian woman who was committed to natural childbirth and
who did not do episiotomies.

I agreed at this point to go to the hospital for pitocin (an
artificial hormone) so that the labor could be started again. I
showered, shampooed, and dried my hair and then ate breakfast.

For all appearances and feelings, I had never begun, let alone completed, the first stage of labor.

The midwife made sandwiches and my husband packed baby clothes. It was snowing lightly as we drove through the city; the rush-hour traffic was over. I certainly didn't feel fully dilated as I calmly gave all my particulars to the admitting clerk and walked upstairs to the maternity unit. I was even able to produce a urine specimen.

Next I was examined by a male obstetrician (whom, we later learned, just happened to be on the floor). He announced that my baby's head was asynclitic (not aligned correctly with the pelvic outlet), and that if it were turned to the right position I could push her out. I understood that he meant a manual rotation—he would turn her head with his hand. As both our vital signs were still normal, there was no hurry and we waited another hour or so for the birth room to become available.

Next, I was given oral prostaglandins to stimulate contractions and an intravenous line was set up for the pitocin drip. I was so preoccupied with watching the IV bottle to make sure there was no added medication that I was jolted by our doctor's voice: "Now you will feel a little prick." A little prick—what for? No one had discussed this with me. I was waiting for the pitocin to go in the IV, and it would take time, maybe hours, for contractions to reestablish. Next I felt a sharp, cold shove of metal in my vagina and the obstetrician said "Push." In total self-defense I PUSHED.

"My god," he said. "You certainly know how to push."

The nurse commented that the baby's heart rate was now at 100. "Push," said the obstetrician again. Bearing down with all my might, I looked at the blank faces of my husband, the general practitioner, and the midwife. Where were my advocates? Realizing that he was yanking out my baby, I pleaded, "Please don't cut me!"

"Push," said the doctor for the third time, snipping an episiotomy, and the baby—Julia—came out. The sole redeeming aspect of this nightmare was that I saw his single hand on the forceps; he hadn't pulled hard on her head.

My husband was frozen speechless throughout. The midwife looked on without a word. My doctor took Julia to a table, suctioned her, and gave her some oxygen. She looked fine to me. I reclined back, stunned at this event which had taken only a matter of moments. "You said I could push the baby out," I protested. "You did," said the obstetrician. "*I just helped you*" (italics mine, in perpetual indignation).

I was still too much in shock to vent my rage. Besides I had to lie still while he stitched up his cruel and unnecessary incision (Julia weighed only six and a half pounds). By now I was nursing Julia and enchanted with her. But soon a primal feeling came up: I've got to get away from here. Now I felt endangered. Our family doctor wanted us to stay; he was concerned about infection, since my membranes had been ruptured for almost four days. I assured him I was not in the least bit sick and if I were going to get an infection, it would happen in the hospital, not at home. (Often, home-birth practitioners who demonstrate independence and autonomy outside the hospital crumble once they are inside it.) I had never planned to have the baby in the hospital; I felt utterly betrayed, and I was determined to leave before another disaster befell me. I was furious that our doctor, whom we had trusted, had abandoned me. He claimed later he had no idea that the obstetrician was going to use forceps—yet he was the one who warned me about the injection of local anesthetic just before.

On the way home we stopped for a take-out lunch and went home to bed. By then we felt only joy and relief for this beautiful, healthy, tranquil little girl who lay between us as we finally dropped off to sleep.

I tried many times to understand the events of my labor. Round and round we went, analyzing, interpreting, reviewing every little detail. I wallowed in every negative emotion— anger, blame, guilt, disappointment—and even tried rationalization. Yet clarity remained out of reach. It was a crushing disappointment, an "immaculate deception." Eleven years later I still feel that the obstetrician was a con artist. He sensed an easy $350, a quick "cut, yank, and sew" job that would permit him to be back to his office in time for his first patient. Obviously he never planned to wait for the pitocin to take effect—and even had the nerve to call later that day and demand payment.

How ironic—when I personally knew so many gentle, wonderful obstetricians—that I should end up with a total stranger who practiced the kind of obstetrics I had warned women against all my professional life. Had I been forewarned I would have chartered a private plane back to Boston.

I thought of all the other problems: snowstorm, airport closed, elevator out of order, no hot water, wrong size catheter, an evil obstetrician—the *random* universe? *Why me?* I agonized.

But one irrefutable point persisted. *I* had stopped my labor, *at home*, without any outside intervention. Why had labor stalled in that way and at that time? For months I asked my colleagues in the natural-birth movement; all were at a loss for explanations and seemed as perplexed by the course of events as I was. This was several months before I met Graham and a couple of years before I attended the ground-breaking first congress of the Pre and Perinatal Psychology Association of North America, in 1983. At that conference, Cheek spoke about his work with patients before delivery to preclude complications arising from their own birth experiences. In my former ignorance, I had not considered the possibility of any such connection.

I came to conclude that there were several facets to the drama of this labor of which I was consciously aware. My own birth was very fast, and I certainly didn't want the same experience for my child. I also didn't want a ruined pelvic floor, which my rapid exit had caused my mother (and I have made it a professional specialty of mine in recompense). I so loved being pregnant and did not want to give up one privileged day of my allotted nine months. I also remember deliberately resisting her arrival on St. Patrick's Day!

I was upset that my husband had left me without a contact number. He hadn't called the night of the bleeding because he thought he might disturb my sleep, yet I was staying up beyond my usual bedtime waiting for his call so I would know how to reach him. Getting more incensed, I remember thinking to myself, "And what if I went into labor and I couldn't contact him? I'm missing my sleep, why doesn't he call? If I went into labor I'd be so tired." In this circle of self-sabotage my anxiety formed a barrier to communication with Julia inside.

I now believe that I sensed his unconscious birth anxiety as he awaited his nonbiological child. In view of Julia's conception by donor insemination, I particularly wanted Geoff to experience her birth and the early bonding phase. Today I know that I went into labor after he left because, unconsciously, I felt safer giving birth without him. In my conscious mind, however, I had the opposite view: that I needed him and the doctor. I thus committed myself to hold everything off until the circumstances were "right"; by not trusting Nature, my instincts backfired. The word I most used when describing Julia's labor was that I felt "abandoned"—by Geoff, our doctor, his midwife. Although they stood there physically, to me they were absent emotionally as my state-dependent memory surfaced during labor. (Interestingly, at my subsequent birth, of my son, under the sun, two male acquaintances who happened to be visiting became my birth attendants, while their wives stayed in the background.)

These insights did not come easily to me. In those days I joined with my colleagues in the view that something just went wrong with the machine, whereas now I appreciate that the body is a report card of a person's consciousness. My humiliating experience with obstetric intervention further stirred me to action. As I heard similar stories in my work I became more empathetic, wondering, as in my own case, what the *reason* was. I had observed that undrugged babies at birth are highly conscious. Although I had never met anyone then who claimed to have relived the experience of birth, I didn't doubt that the memory of such an event is recorded somewhere and somehow. In my case, however, I was sure that there was no need for *me* to relive my own fast, easy birth because I couldn't see any connection with Julia's birth.

I later learned that there were influences during the first two trimesters of my gestation that shaped my personality, my life, and my labor with Julia. But this meant taking a huge leap into the unknown, going way beyond my formal education, to consider that memory would be possible for a tiny embryo—and even individual cells like a sperm and an egg.

CHAPTER THREE

The Links Between Brain, Mind, and Memory

Memory is an essential component of self, learning, thinking, intelligence and communication. I propose that we consider them inseparable and treat the whole cluster as a human endowment that is innate rather than developmental.

—DAVID B. CHAMBERLAIN

An understanding of how memory works is central to any endeavor that explores recalled experiences from prenatal life, particularly in a world that is skeptical of such early memory. New theories about preverbal memory do not fit the traditional models of the brain and mind; such memories have been typically dismissed as "fantasies." But the view that memory begins with sensory functions and consciousness beginning after birth is dying, albeit slowly.

All memory involves three steps: perception, storage, and retrieval. Perceptions are stored in different places in the body, in the biochemical structure of cells, but as Ronald Melzack wrote in an article on phantom limbs, "We do not need a body to feel a body."

Today, the brain can no longer be seen as a control box in the skull, a kind of tape recorder with a segmental system of neural pathways reaching throughout the body. Likewise, memory storage can no longer be considered an exclusive province of the various parts of the brain. In fact, it has never been determined where and how the brain stores memories.

THE FLUID BRAIN

A modern view is that memory has no location, no fixed content in the brain, but rather that the brain has frames of reference or maps that serve in a selective process of categorization. It is not the contents of experience that are encoded in memory but organizational patterns that process experience in certain ways. The brain can repeat any of its former reactions, because memories are part of the cellular chemistry of the body, specifically protein synthesis.

The nervous, endocrine, and immune systems are all reciprocally connected through fluid pathways. The brain is a gland, too, because it produces hormones, contains receptors for hormones, and is awash in hormones. Genes, molecules, behavior, and emotion are all tied together. These chemical bonds, stated Janov, "are every bit as strong as the chain links on an anchor." Variable interactions can alter the way genes are expressed, and lead to both structural and functional changes in the brain. Thus the nervous system is everywhere; it is a system of liquefied information flowing through the body! And the unconscious mind includes energy cycles and biological rhythms as well as innate and genetic characteristics.

There are over 100 substances that activate and organize interactions between genes and the environment. Chemical mediators called neurotransmitters allow nerve cells to interact with each other. There are two levels: the "hardware" of the anatomical structure and the "software" of hormones and substances that bathe those structures in all kinds of messages. These informational substances can be signaled across very different compartments of the body and over widely varying time periods. As well as neurotransmitters, there are substances made by endocrine glands (hormones) and the immune system (cytokines or immunotransmitters). Such chemical messengers transmit, receive, and monitor the flow of information throughout the body, but more slowly than the direct transmission of information through the anatomical nervous system.

The same chemicals that influence mood in the brain control the integrity of the body. Neuropeptides direct the movement of key components in the immune system. These monocytes— a specific form of white blood cell essential in wound healing —are produced in bone marrow, but they can become glial cells that support nervous tissue in the brain. They are believed to move back and forth in the body, having been programmed in the brain.

When experience is encoded under the influence of mood-altering drugs, for example, the memory becomes "statebound" or dependent on that same condition. As a result, the memory is lost when the drug is out of a person's system, but regained when it is readministered. Similarly, physiological states of fear and anxiety can be induced with certain drugs, just as rapid shallow breathing (often taught to pregnant women) causes the same feeling of anxiety, as does involuntary hyperventilation. Breathing practices affect consciousness through the presence of neuropeptides in the brain, too.

Our potential for adaptation to different environmental stimuli is diverse, and adaptation occurs via these chemical substances to bind experiences in state-dependent ways, as just described. These psychobiological states are myriad, including thirst, hunger, sexual feelings, and—of course—significant experiences about birth that encompass fear, pain, and stress. As the unborn baby develops, connections form between nerve cells in a basic human structure as well as in an individual and variable way, according to personal experiences. High concentrations of hormones and/or neurotransmitters during critical periods of brain development can permanently affect metabolism, growth, reproduction, information processing, behavior, and immunity. These substances control the brain's participation in the neuro-endocrine-immune systems and co-determine the responsiveness of their own central nervous controllers. Hence, they create the range of function and tolerance of their own feedback control systems throughout life.

IMPRINTING

In 1973 the Nobel Prize was awarded to Konrad Lorenz for the discovery of imprinting—very fast, single-event learning that happens during a time of extreme stress or transition. Lorenz discovered that when he was the first contact for newly hatched goslings, they bonded with him as a substitute mother. There are certain stages in human development, too—especially prenatally and immediately postpartum—when the potential for a powerful imprint or engram is at a peak.

During times of emotional, physical, chemical, or surgical stress, hormones and other messenger substances in the body are released and imprint an experience in a way that makes it bound to that specific stressful state, influencing various systems to encode a memory in a special manner. A traumatic event remains deeply imprinted as organic memory, but the accompanying shock creates a neurochemical barrier of repression between the unconscious and conscious mind.

Many traits, personality characteristics, and physiological predispositions develop as a result of the intrauterine environment and determine what aspects will manifest in an individual's genetic composition. Janov points out that we are discussing a "biological reality, not a psychological metaphor." Stress during pregnancy can be as much a cause of imbalance within the body's systems as iodine deficiency or cocaine abuse. The fetus senses his mother's altered hormone output, over-active pulse, or high blood pressure, but he experiences the consequences, not the cause. Clues may come later in life if connections are made in a state-dependent way. (We tend to regress under stress.) Often the adult learns that the negative experience had nothing to do with him, but a fetus is not able to discriminate and he may have carried undue feelings of guilt, responsibility, or rejection ever since. Imprints influence perceptions and personality development; they do not fade with the passage of time.

Thus, in altered states of consciousness, such as hypnosis or primal therapy, the stress hormones can be reactivated so that the "information" that was bound in that emotional state can be brought through associative connections into consciousness. Anecdotal accounts of birth and prenatal memories are impressive and are increasing. Obviously there has to be memory, or there is a dilemma in claiming that we relive something that never entered consciousness or even antedated its very existence! Rank reminded us of the homing instincts of birds of passage and migrating fish, which return to "*their place of birth from every strange place to which they have been taken or to which they themselves have migrated*" (italics his).

Psychosomatic symptoms and regression phenomena are manifestations of the same dynamics as state-dependent learning and behavior. Altered levels of arousal and emotion are responsible for both the encoding and the later recall of stress-related problems in altered states of consciousness. In this context, the absolute prohibition of a single drink by Alcoholics Anonymous makes sense; one drink may be enough to activate the physiological systems and create the memory-state again.

PRENATAL DEVELOPMENT

Skeptics who focus on the anatomical brain and nervous system argue that the further back we go in prenatal memory, the less "material" there is to account for that memory. Preverbal and precognitive memory, they say, could not happen before the development of the cortex of the brain, which works like a computer drawing on networks of myelinated nerves. But as we have seen from the new theories, memory is not limited by anatomy or myelin, and communication in the nervous system is far more complex than just nerve conduction. According to Montagu, the triune division of the brain into its developmental components 1) brainstem, 2) limbic system, and 3) neocortex is not only simplistic but "anatomically and physiologically unsound."

We have discussed a current model of brain processes that explains memory and learning as a form of selection. This selection, as we have seen, is dependent on the state of the organism. Therefore, adaptive patterns that were stimulated and imprinted during birth act as a frame of reference for organizing and interpreting later experiences in life. Before and after birth, patterns of response tend to become fixed and are selected habitually, in ways that are learned by a particular person in his or her own environment. Transformed physical feelings thus become "a fixed part of our psychological anatomy," concluded Mott, and "the original capacity to feel is not increased by experience but divided by experience." At the core of all these feelings lies the tightly compacted group of prenatal feelings that affect our reactions. In fact, as Chamberlain wrote, "birth-related fears and disturbed behavior are a type of learning where the memory is enshrined in the symptoms."

BIRTH MEMORIES

Evidence of birth memory, especially associated with trauma, has been reported frequently in the last seventy years, beginning with Rank in 1929. Rank noted that Freud had a patient whose complaints "that the world seemed to him disguised by a veil" could be traced back to his birth in a caul (unruptured membranes). Freud saw the problem of perinatal memory as "the most ticklish of the whole analytic doctrine," but accepted Groddeck's insistence that "what we can call Ego behaves essentially passively in life, and that . . . we are 'lived' by unknown and uncontrollable forces."

In *Babies Remember Birth*, Chamberlain presented reports by his clients that included family secrets, rude remarks, and even physical abuse—matters that were surely concealed from the child after birth. He found that birth memories were distinctly personal, original, and uninfluenced by others, yet they had inner consistency, held up over time, and contained both facts not consciously known and technical details of labor and delivery not expected from lay persons. There was often astute criticism of how the birth was managed!

Almost all of the pioneers in pre- and perinatal psychology were forced to accommodate the idea of prenatal memory—often with great personal resistance. Convinced clients and verifiable stories obliged these therapists to change their frameworks to incorporate concepts of increasingly earlier awareness. Not infrequently there was evidence such as a reappearance of bruises or pressure marks from forceps, or even breath odor of anesthetic gas. Furthermore, going back to birth and earlier yielded better therapeutic results than, as Cheek noted, "letting patients climb around the branches of memory and getting nowhere at the top of the tree of life."

As a result, progressive psychotherapists now firmly believe that no satisfactory exploration or integration can be completed until it reaches the earliest levels of the mind because, as Fodor pointed out, it is before birth that the psychic foundation of our being is laid. Traditional frameworks clearly must be changed to incorporate the idea of awareness at the very origin of life.

Recall of events as early as first-trimester attempted abortions and loss of a twin are increasingly common, and in many cases have been confirmed by the mother. Canadian psychologist Andrew Feldmar, as well as researchers at Loyola University in Chicago, found that some adults would attempt suicide at the same time each year. These attempts turned out to be related to the month in which the mother had tried to terminate the pregnancy. The survivors also had used a method of suicide similar to the mother's abortion attempt—for example, instruments or chemicals.

Graham relived an attempt by his mother to abort him, and when he telephoned her with his insight, she exclaimed, "How could you have known? I never even told your father."

THE MANY LEVELS
OF THE MIND

We embody our defense through our muscular system in a manner that Wilhelm Reich called *armoring*. Less well known is Norwegian psychologist Lillemor Johnsen's theory about insufficient muscle tone: muscles that became flaccid rather than tense. Lisbeth Marcher and Erik Jarlness in Denmark followed her path and suggested that tendons and fascia store the prebirth memories, whereas postnatal issues are more associated with muscles. When a person is regressed to birth and before, some of the primitive birth reflexes that were lost in infancy reappear. Likewise, Vladimir Raikov's research with hypnosis showed that adults could be regressed to early infancy and recover authentic neurological reflexes, as well as behavior and brain wave activity characteristic of that period of development.

Memory comes from the Greek word for "to care for"; Boadella suggested that all our experiences need to be digested and "cared for." His framework of the three layers of embryological structure helps to integrate the concepts of mind, body, soul, thought, emotion, and gut response. The outer layer, or surface, of the skin constitutes what Mott called "fetal skin feeling"— impressions from the uterus and how the infant was handled after birth. The eye and ear are specialized developments from this ectoderm. Kinesthetic affect is the flow of feeling associated with movements in the middle layer (mesoderm), and the umbilical affect is the flow of feeling associated with the sense of life and energy being pumped into the center of one's body through the umbilical cord (the endoderm or inner layer). Likewise, three energy fields are generated that organize the embryonic layers and the "streams of affect" that are felt in each one: the endoderm field, which is emotional and the "gut stream"; the ectoderm layer, which is mental and the "thought stream"; and the mesoderm, wherein one finds the muscle stream, and "vital component." "Emotional expression is a total organismic event in which the muscular system, the visceral system, and the ideational system are all simultaneously involved," concluded Boadella in his book *Lifestreams.*

The ego, as a form of subjective perception, determines the interaction between the self and the outside world—the relationship between thoughts and external physical reality. Boadella explained that every ego state reflects a bodily attitude, and every character expression has a physiological anchoring: "tension patterns of the body are a person's frozen history. . . . Mind is outside the body and body is inside the mind." What connects all of this to pre- and perinatal psychology is the idea that a person's identity originates in the physiological relationship between mother and child—what Chilton Pearce called the "mother matrix."

WHAT ARE THE LINKS BETWEEN BRAIN, MEMORY, AND MIND?

Amazingly, it is possible to stimulate the brain when patients are conscious, and even to remove a whole hemisphere without loss of awareness, perceptions, or memory. People who anatomically lack a neocortex have graduated from college! We certainly don't need a cortex to react with a visceral response —fear, rage, and other emotions—to painful stimuli. Indeed, there are primary survival mechanisms in the ancient structures of our nervous system that have served us well through time.

Jung proposed the concept of a collective unconscious of archetypical primal forms whose "vividness originated at a time when the unconscious did not yet think, but perceived." His theory has been very useful in explaining the common themes of myths and dreams, as we will see in the next chapter.

Fodor suggested that:

While we can trace the beginnings of the conscious mind, we know nothing of the beginnings of the unconscious, for if the unconscious mind exists in the pre-natal state and if we admit its existence, we might have to face questions as to its function.

All repetitive acts give evidence of memory. We cannot imagine the function of our autonomic internal systems without postulating an organic memory that not only registers the process of growth but also reacts to dangers that threaten the organism. The unconscious mind of each of us is in complete possession of all the data that concern the body. As Edger Cayce stated: "Mind is the builder, spirit is the life, and the physical is the result."

PRENATAL ORIGIN OF SYMPTOMS: THE CHAIN OF EVIDENCE FOR EARLY AWARENESS AND MEMORY

The history of psychotherapy, according to hypnotherapist Ernest Rossi, co-author with David Cheek of *Mind-Body Therapy*, could be summarized as an "effort to understand the amnesia surrounding the origins of psychological problems." These problems always have physical manifestations, because the mind and body are intertwined. Likewise, Mott explained that psychological feeling derives from older physical feeling; the earlier the physical experience, the more likely it is to create emotions. This deeper memory, explained Cheek, is less flawed than ordinary memory and exists despite assaults on consciousness, injury, anesthesia, and stress. The shock of birth, with its sudden flooding of our senses, destroys the mechanism of that prenatal consciousness but it lives on in the "feelings of the organs."

There is a parallel for prenatal amnesia in postnatal repression and infantile amnesia, which extend from birth until about five years of age—the stage of ego development. Thereafter, thoughts and consciously held feelings predominate. Mott believed that, after ages five to seven, physical experiences only reanimate earlier existing ones.

In Mott's scheme, an organ of the body may evoke feeling but later lose that power through repression. However, those feelings can be transferred to another organ and appear as "unconscious" feelings to the new organ. Each time the "affect" changes its position, the consciousness of the completed stage *becomes* feeling, without direct consciousness, while at the same time the new stage awakens a new experience of conscious awareness to which all earlier stages appear as psychological feeling.

Mott further explained that the distinction between the conscious and unconscious mind is at root a division between neural feelings (after ages five to seven) and earlier "blood feelings." These early feelings derive from the circulation between fetus, placenta, and umbilical cord—the "total uterine organism" which comprises the original "mind-making apparatus." Mott considered the universal pattern of the nucleus and periphery as "the two great primal categories." In human development he designates the fetal skin as the organ of nuclear feeling and the placenta as the organ of peripheral feeling. The umbilical cord is the organ of synthesis between the two poles, linking them by a two-way flow. This system tunes the unborn child to cosmic rhythms and develops his sense of a space-time structure. As further examples of this basic configuration of nucleus and periphery, Mott pointed to the solar system, the living cell, and the atom.

Within the uterus, the nucleus-ego-fetus is symbolically forever being drawn into the periphery (placenta) "destroyed there, renewed and restored." The fetus experiences a "dynamic sense of thrust and penetrating power" via the arteries, but becomes "hollow and victim" in relation to the returning venous blood. The periphery thus heightens, protects, and threatens the nuclear sense. Although there are no nerves in the cord, "the beat of blood evokes those primary elements of feeling which form the basis of mind." The umbilical circulation modulates the nuclear feeling of the fetus by constantly interrelating it with the peripheral feeling offered by the functions of the placenta.

ENERGY AND FIELDS OF RESONANCE

Groddeck reminded us that the expression so constantly used—"the forces of nature"—shows us that since humankind began to think, we have known as modern physics has proved, that all is energy.

> There is nothing but energy, pouring through us, and working in us, and in it we are immersed. . . . Energy follows thought. . . . The ideas of leading thinkers assume a mental form, when the quality of desire begins to enter in and there is an emotional reaction to the thoughts which the ideas have evoked and the form is gradually built. Thus the work goes on and the energy of the soul and of the mind and of the desire correlate with the energy of matter, and a definite form comes into being.

Rupert Sheldrake put forth a hypothesis in 1981 that memory is inherent throughout nature and demonstrates "habits" rather than laws. Memory is transmitted from one generation to the next by a process of "morphic resonance." The formative morphic, or "M," fields make it easier for knowledge of previous generations to be learned than new information. Recent experiments support this theory: real Morse code was learned faster than a phony version, and crossword puzzles were easier to solve if they had been previously solved by other people.

In animals, telepathic transmission of danger is an important survival mechanism. In humans, telepathy is a depth of communication of thoughts by methods beyond the scope of our five senses which serves the infant until verbal skills develop. Far from being a spiritual or metaphysical manifestation, it has been shown to be mediated by certain areas of brain cells.

Communication is possible in this way between humans, animals, and plants.

SPIRIT AND MATTER

Divine consciousness makes its presence felt in different spheres of human awareness and behavior—mental, sensory, and physical. Illumination is not only psychological but also physiological, observed Groddeck. There is a momentum toward wholeness in us all, toward the expression of our spirit's longing to harmoniously interact with whom we have soul connections.

Radhakrishnan explained that all forms veil a divine thought, idea, or truth and are the tangible manifestation of a divine concept. Alice Bailey suggested that in meditation we try to receive "impresses of the higher self" directly into the physical brain via the mind. In the higher state of contemplation, we open up to receive into the physical brain "that which the *soul itself perceives* as it looks outward upon those new fields of perception, and sees and knows without the use of imagination or reason."

Peerbolte proposed that the inner self belongs to the egg's quality, related to an "I-function"—an original part of the egg, even existing in the ovarial state. The spiritual self, he felt, was invisible within the field of attraction between the sperm and egg. Similar to Mott, he believed that the center of the personality later on becomes related to the carbon dioxide and oxygen balance in the womb, an idea that is central to William Hull's definition of the prenatal suffocation syndrome.

Ideas about space and time are inborn categories of the intrauterine state. Swedish anthropologist Tore Håkansson likewise pointed out that cavities and round forms must be the earliest kinesthetic or body-sense experiences representing perception of the uterus. In the West we have forgotten the significance of the navel as the place through which life entered, the "entrance and exit, the connecting link." He reminded us that in the East, the navel is recognized as the center of biological and psychological functions, which are experienced as total unity in the womb: "After birth comes the separation, of an outside world leading to the artificial division of mind and body—mankind's [sic] age old riddle."

What physicists call matter and what mystics call spirit may be different levels of vibration of one's own fundamental energy—the watershed between body and soul. The question Boadella asked is, Does the world of matter generate invisible fields or do the invisible fields generate the world of matter? Eastern pundits have considered matter as energy in its densest or lowest form, and spirit as this same energy in its highest or most subtle form; matter is spirit descending and spirit is matter ascending.

Jung defined spirit as the living body seen from within; the body is the outer manifestation of the living spirit, the two really being one. Laing pragmatically remarked that "it seems to me to be strictly impossible to tell, from the observation of someone dying, whether mind, soul or spirit is extinguished as the brain dies, or whether he, she, it, or they vacate the brain and body."

Groddeck believed that life is positive electricity or spirit, and substance is negative electricity or matter. Life is the father and begets; substance is the mother and conceives. The third aspect he postulated is active energy, the resultant interaction of life and sustenance called consciousness, or soul. This is the same triangle as Father, Son, and Spirit or Holy Ghost.

BEYOND THE BODY

The phenomena of out-of-body experiences and past lives, while not the focus of this book, certainly belong in any discussion of memory. In an article titled "The Outer Limits of Memory," Chamberlain pointed out that scientific ridicule and indifference to evidence for expanded consciousness and birth, womb, and past-life memory have delayed discovery of who we really are.

Cheek documented a case in which an adult under hypnosis described his mother's dress during pregnancy (a dress he could never have seen because she had given it away before the birth). How does the unborn baby inside know what is outside? Cheek felt that the mechanism is telepathy, such as we see in young animals that sense a signal of danger from their mother and remain absolutely silent. Fodor had already considered that telepathy may be an additional channel of awareness open to the child in addition to sense perceptions and, like Cheek, he believed that telepathic impressions from mother to child remain imbedded in some manner in his developing unconscious.

Researchers such as Grof, Raymond Moody, Brian Weiss, Kenneth Ring, and Ian Stephenson have explored past lives, out-of-body experiences, ancestral memories, certain archetypal experiences, and awareness of a "universal mind" or "cosmic consciousness." Most of these investigators are medical doctors, and they raise the prospect of some form of nonphysical memory. The brain may work like a tuning device and storage may be outside both the brain and the body. Out-of-body events are experienced while the brain resides firmly in its skull, and memory endures when cells do not. Much of the evidence of such events comes from cardiovascular surgeons and emergency-room physicians who resuscitate patients.

Plentiful anecdotes of past-life memory exist, and Professor Ian Stephenson, MD, of the University of Virginia, has documented with satisfactory verification many cases among Americans. He has also thoroughly researched the literature in other cultures, particularly India. Yet no one knows what the connection is between the physical structures of a brain and a body that existed in another period of time.

In confronting the question of whether the mind can survive the death of the physical brain, Candace Pert, of the National Institutes of Health, considered both quantum physics and information theory. Subatomic physics has blown away such concepts as space, time, cause, and effect. In physical equations, things can collapse up and down, she explains, so it's possible that this information storage could reconfigure and transform itself into some other reality.

Artificial boundaries between memory, learning, communication, and personality—like those between mind and body or psychology and neurology—may be no more than "illusions of convenience." A reductionistic approach has set these disciplines apart for purposes of study and (mis)education. Instead, Chamberlain has suggested that memory is "an innate and ageless endowment of human consciousness which spans all time periods."

Birth and Prenatal Symbolism in Dreams and Myths

Myths come from where the heart is, and where the experience is, even as the mind may wonder why people believe these things.
—JOSEPH CAMPBELL

No study of prenatal and perinatal experiences would be complete without looking at dreams,* myths, legends, and their universal symbols of the uterine period and birth. Birth images and symbols flourish in the nine-tenths of our being that lie beyond the narrow limits of our conscious mind. The same symbols continually appear in fantasies, dreams, myths, and legends (primal ocean, tree of life, animal sacrifice). One writer even complained of the "monotony of fundamental ideas!"

Symbolism is a soundless, universal language that includes biological functions and complex transcendental realities, and it shows up even in dreams of children, uneducated persons, and neurotic and psychotic patients. We inherit this ancient symbolism of feelings, but we have no direct contact with those feelings. As commonplace examples, many people are afraid of tunnels, caves, and elevators, or they dislike turtleneck

---

* I noticed when reviewing Silberer's articles that the German word for dream, *Traum*, is almost the same as both the English and German word for *trauma*. In the second edition of the *Oxford English Dictionary*, Kluge says that the English word dream comes from the old English drēam or the West German *Draum*. He suggests that the origin is the same Greek root, *thrylos*, meaning noise or a din. And the uterus in which we grew was a place of considerable, constant noise in which the fetus spends much of his time in a dream state.

sweaters, scarves, neckties, and hats—and don't know why.

In fact, dreams were the earliest proof of prenatal consciousness and memory, predating hypnosis and psychotherapy by millennia. Something in the mind desires healing and sees to it that at the proper time the right material is brought forth in dreams and associations. Fodor called this integrative design principle the soul or higher self, and he suggested that "a partnership develops between the patient's conscious and unconscious mind, serving the mysterious purposes of the latter without full comprehension on the part of the former."

MYTH

Joseph Campbell, the renowned mythologist, explained that myths present the "challenging persistent suggestion of more remaining to be experienced than will ever be known or told," and that "the logic, heroes and deeds of myths survive into modern times." The same images in primitive rituals often turn up on the analyst's couch, and the modern witch doctor is the psychoanalyst versed in the lore and language of dreams.

Jung's theory of archetypes described forms or images of a collective nature that occur throughout the world as a constituent of myths and at the same time as self-generated individual products of unconscious origin. Both Freudian imagery and Jung's archetypes have their roots in prenatal experiences, and prenatal dynamics are the root of all postnatal feelings. Until very recently, however, psychoanalysts (with the exception of Rank, Mott, Fodor, and Peerbolte) did not extend their analysis to before birth. But the infantile character of dreams and myths goes much further back and has a much deeper basis than was previously admitted.

Freud recognized "the myth of the birth of the hero" as the nucleus of myth formation. Great heroes of antiquity are endless travelers. They have to overcome difficulties of an incredible nature en route to inaccessible destinations. Often the hero is carried in the belly of a fish, dragon, sea serpent, or whale. Significantly, if he does find the way to return, his fate is sealed by death, so the quest to find a new life by rebirth is allegorical.

The hero represents the type who tries to overcome, first, a severe birth trauma by a compensatory repetition of it in his deeds. And so in the subsequent (infantile) wish fantasies, the hero is regularly cut from his mother's womb. Heroic invulnerability is thus explained as a kind of "permanent uterus" that the hero brings with him into the world as armor, horny skin, or helmet (magic hood).

The second trauma is weaning, which is often linked with exposure to and interactions with animals who may mother and nurse the fetal hero, such as Romulus and Remus. "Authentic reminiscences of the two experienced primal traumas," Fodor concluded, "are at the bottom of myths exactly as they are of neuroses."

Laing poetically summarized the major prenatal and birth themes in myths and legends in his book *The Facts of Life*. (See Glossary at the back of this book for the meanings of any unfamiliar terms.)

LEGENDARY SYMBOL	BIOLOGICAL FOUNDATION
In many myths,	
the hero	zygote
is put in a container of some kind	
a boat	zona pellucida
a box	
a sphere	
a casket	
into a river	uterine canal/tube/duct
or the sea	
lands on the shore	endometrium
is saved	little understood adoption
and nurtured by	of the blastocyst by the

LEGENDARY SYMBOL	BIOLOGICAL FOUNDATION
animals or lowly people	uterine endometrium
prospers	and
becomes adopted by	grows into a fetus
the King and Queen	in
of the city	womb city
	until
leaves	birth
finds after many adventures	and subsequent adventures
his real parents	in correlating M_0 with M_1, M_2

(Note: M_o, M_1, and M_2 refer to the mother before conception, after conception, and after birth.)

Prenatal Nostalgia and Symbolic Return

Déjà vu is often prenatal nostalgia. Speaking from personal experience, Fodor explained that "visions bound up with earliest memories are not connected with any earthly experience, but something I had left rather than somewhere I was going or could hope to go." Lake agreed that many an adult has an intuitive feeling that there was a time early in the womb when he did not need to earn security—it was a right. Boadella called this fetal life of the closed center "cosmosis."

Fetal nostalgia appears as a fascination for mysteries, cave exploration, submarine research, space travel, voyages of discovery, the lure of faraway islands, or the desire to climb unconquered mountain peaks. Along with the typical dreams of a prenatal royal estate is the childhood fantasy of being a foundling, with real parents somewhere of high lineage to help the child claim his lost heritage. Dreams of getting to a train and having the gate shut in the dreamer's face, or a broken bridge, or being stuck in an exam situation represent a frustrated return.

Alleged UFO abductions are often fantasies or hallucinations of pre- and perinatal events. According to an article in the *Journal of Psychohistory*, individuals who claimed to have been plucked up from the earth and taken into a spaceship were often Cesarean born. In contrast, the vaginally born ascended a rope or ladder to the placenta-shaped craft.

Many burial customs reveal the belief that we pass away by the same path through which we come into life. In some tribes the dead have been doubled up for burial in the fetal posture, laid out on islands and mountaintops, or even sent out to sea in boats. These gestures accommodate the wish to return to the womb after death.

Initiation rites provide ceremonies of rebirth, such as the enforced seclusion of puberty rites. The deeper we descend on the scale of civilization, observed Fodor, the more importance is attached to an allegorical return to the womb as assurance of the reality of a new life.

Fodor proposed in his book *Search for the Beloved* that belief in a future life springs from the certainty of a past existence, "the haunting glamor of which forever escapes clear recollection but remains as obscure organismic memories."

Dreams

Sleep researchers tell us that we dream from three to five times each night, and that dreams occur at intervals of every hour to an hour and a half. Rapid eye movement (REM), which indicates dreaming, begins before birth. From research done on preterm infants, it would seem that most of their sleep is REM after twenty-three weeks.

Nietzsche observed that in our sleep and in our dreams we pass through:

the whole thought of earlier humanity. . . . In the same way that man reasons in his dreams he reasoned when in the

waking state many thousands of years ago. . . . The dream
carries us back into earlier states of human culture, and af-
fords us a means of understanding it better.

Myths have a unitary source that also is the source of the
dream. For Campbell, dream was "personalized myth" and myth
was the "depersonalized dream." Both myth and dream are
symbolic in the same general way of the dynamics of the psyche.
But in a dream "the forms are quirked by the peculiar troubles
of the dreamer, whereas in myth the problem and solutions
shown are directly valid for all mankind." In the case of prenatal
experiences we find universal symbols, but in specific constel-
lations to reflect the quality of uterine life.

Freud pointed out that "sleep is a re-activation of the intrauterine situation. We have rest, warmth, and absence of
stimuli." Many people sleep in the fetal position, and threshold
birth symptoms may be expressed in the frequent twitching of
the legs on going to sleep. (Restless foot syndrome is also seen
in the waking state; I know an obstetrician whose foot-tapping
during a conversation is incessant.) Rank believed that dreams
universally express either the desire to reenter the mother's
womb or anxiety at the inability to do so.

Fodor was aware that studying the dreams that precede and
follow delivery can be instructive. Expectations around labor
and birth tend to mobilize the fear of falling; induce nightmares
of water, fire, and suffocation; and may even produce symptoms
of claustrophobia. Nightmares of mothers fleeing from pursuit
(to escape the ordeal of birth) may alternate with erotic dreams
in which a newborn son figures as a lover (during intercourse),
according to Fodor.

Calvin Hall studied 590 unselected dreams and found that
60 percent of them showed overt pre- and perinatal images—
in nonpregnant subjects. In her book *Pregnancy and Dreams*,
Patricia Maybruck analyzed 1,048 dreams of pregnant women
and discovered that 70 percent were negative. Four hundred
five of the dreams were nightmares from which women awoke
terrified and upset. Another 30 percent contained anxiety-

producing elements; hostile or threatening characters; environmental disasters such as storms, earthquakes, and fires; or deaths and funerals. Unfortunately, the author apparently never read Rank, Fodor, or Mott, because she failed to interpret a single one of those dreams as the mother's prenatal imprints! Maybruck has tips for pregnant women to "control" their dreams, but as Campbell reminds us, "symbols of mythology are not manufactured; they cannot be ordered and most significantly, they cannot be permanently suppressed."

Of course, dreams are infinite in meaning and their interpretation is infinitely arguable. For example, fear or any other emotion in a dream may be retrojection from the higher levels of the mind back to the prenatal foundation, or it may be an actual mobilization of deeply buried, organic memories. Dreams betray the details of uterine life and repeat the birth trauma in typical ways. The conscious understanding of these prenatal symbols can have therapeutic value. Peerbolte, for example, reported the case of a woman who had migraine headaches from the fantasy of being in an animal's jaws. These abated when the patient connected the image with her birth trauma. A woman who carried a deceased twin alongside the living one for the last ten weeks of her pregnancy had a constantly recurring dream. She saw her dead baby in a car, sinking into a lake, and she couldn't open any window for him to get out. Visible relief swept across her face by my suggestions that the car/lake images symbolized the uterus and the window represented the birth canal.

Structure of the Dream

Usually in dreams about pre- and perinatal events, the dreamer is alone. Until very recently, any companion was thought to relate to the placenta. This was before ultrasound technology revealed the vanishing twin phenomenon. Today we know that a high percentage of twins are lost in the uterus, and there are many survivors who indeed had a human companion in the uterus.* Dreams of the placenta are far more universal, however.

Most dreams have a hidden date or in some way reveal the period of life into which the events of the dream fit. In the prenatal period, there may be clues from the ratio of body (especially head) size to the surroundings: the larger the space, the smaller the baby.

The dreamer always knows the meaning of his or her dreams, but may be unable to bring this knowledge into the conscious mind. Mott believed that dreams function as a link between the two systems operating in the human psyche, thought and feelings. When we awaken and remember a dream, we are really remembering the old context of the feelings rather than conceptual wholes into which they have become integrated. But we cannot express the old context of the feelings, for the conscious mind knows nothing of it. Resistance is not an exclusive manifestation of the conscious mind, and inhibition of association or recollection can be part of the dream process, as with any other regressive experience.

The dream mind makes no half-statements. If a person dreams of an escape, the nature of the danger from which he or she is escaping will also be present, concealed in the same dream, or emerge during a discussion of the dream. The dream mind often likes a play of opposites and so events are often reversed: Birth can be either climbing up a ladder or falling down a hole. Names may be spelled backwards or appear in the form of acronyms like Derma, for "dear ma." The unconscious enjoys puns—for example, a mailbox for a vagina!

Dreams tell only one story, according to Mott, here a piece and there a piece, which in total is the story of the "evocation of the pattern of the feelings in the womb and their migration

---

* Perhaps nonliterate societies knew that intuitively which would explain the universal ritual of disposing of the placenta in variously prescribed ways. Even today, many ethnic groups will refuse to go into modern health care facilities to give birth, for fear that they will not be allowed to have the placenta and bury it according to their cultural imperative.

and transformation through the postnatal body." It is the persistence of the same context in dream after dream that ultimately yields the proof, explained Mott, when the "outward form of the dream often belies its hidden consistency." The more complex the mosaic becomes, the easier it is for its possessor to find in dreams an immediate meaning; and the same applies to myths, fantasies, fairy tales, and all manner of collective symbols.

SYMBOLISM

The repetition of symbols over time allows them to stand as an image or picture for something else. Symbols are not invented. They are there—part of the "inalienable state of man," as in Jung's archetypes of the collective unconscious. Campbell pointed out that, "indeed one might say that all conscious thought and action are the unavoidable consequence of unconscious symbolization, that mankind is animated by the symbol."

Of course, every birth symbol can lend itself to a variety of interpretations other than birth. Jacob's ladder, for example, can symbolize the journey to rebirth (reversed) or the cord connecting Jacob to a maturing placenta. Some dream experts recommend picking out nouns and verbs to decipher the message. Others emphasize finding the most emotional element in the dream: feelings recognize no analogy, only identity.

Symbols of Sexuality

A woman's flowers symbolize virginity; by the same token we have the old-fashioned term *defloration*. (I know of an obstetrician who routinely cuts an episiotomy on all her patients and then she gives each one a flower.)

Sexual feelings are often expressed in dreams by the playing of musical instruments or flying. A ring and finger may represent vagina and penis. The penis is sometimes symbolized by a thumb or a "wooden leg," which sounds humorous, but to the fetus it may be an experience of internal crushing, as in rape, perhaps later followed by external crushing in birth. Fear of rape may originate in the fear of birth by a translation of the crushing experience at birth through her mother's genitals onto a woman's own genital tract. Parental intercourse is also symbolized as an earthquake, tempest, or invading war. Adults have recalled fetal experiences of great pressure and discomfort while their parents engaged in intercourse during late pregnancy in the "missionary position."

Fodor related an amusing joke: Two embryos were talking about the future and what they planned to be. "I shall become a lawyer because lawyers can always defend themselves," said one. The other replied, "I shall be a prizefighter so I can take a smack at the guy who comes in every night and spits in my eye."

Birth through the vagina can be evaluated in terms of intercourse and may arouse incestuous feelings. The original sin, according to Fodor, means incest, and our sense of it began in the womb—entering mother as father and being born of her as self. Father-castration fantasies arise from the prenatal trauma of passing through and being separated from the mother's genitals. Usually the vagina is denied in myths and fairy tales, which, as we have seen already, is due to repression of the birth trauma experienced there. As a result, there is a "vaginal bypass"—the hero is cut from the womb—which is happening literally more and more with today's growing Cesarean rate.

Symbols of Conception

All prenatal states cause a regression toward conception, according to Peerbolte's speculations. The ovarian state is often symbolized in dreams by communities: when a relation to the "terrible mother" has to be expressed, these communities become "communists" or "concentration camps."

Oceanic dreams, or dreams of cosmic feelings which are preconceptual and unbounded, represent conception. In contrast, the image of a breakwater points to fertilization. Conception may be represented by lightning or fire (which is also a symbol of birth). Airplanes and "little men from another planet" are symbols for sperm. The vase represents the egg; it receives the spirit. This is an ancient symbol, an archetype, for the Holy Grail. Silberer, in 1912, gave examples of sperm dreams and believed them to be the wish to go back into the father's body. Campbell related a ritual among African bushmen that symbolizes the sperm journey in all its detail, from the crowd experience to traveling up the mucus channels to gamete death and rebirth as a zygote. Stephen Seely, at the University of Manchester Medical School, suggests that about one percent of published dreams can be recognized as representing some phase of gamete development. He interpreted as sperm memories a set of dreams of evisceration or dissection of the legs and or pelvis. In the testicles, when the primitive spermatogonia are developing into spermatids, they lose almost all their entire cytoplasm, the mature sperm being mainly nucleus and a slender tail (flagellum.) The phase at first when the dreamer is dead may refer to the state before motility, and in a dream of Freud himself, he described a long journey in a cab through a town and then a mountainous landscape.

Dreams of stalagmites or pillars of different sizes surrounding the dreamer who is unable to make herself heard could be interpreted as the primitive oogonia developing in the ovary. One winner ripens on a narrow stalk, and after its release the rest of the maturing follicles shrivel up. Seely speculates that dreams of sorting objects such as cutlery, trinkets, pairs hint at chromosome division.

The new being that springs from the egg and the sperm cannot retain both sexual components. "The lost sexual potential has not been extinguished but retires underground to haunt the winner for the rest of its life," warned Fodor: "Some of the deepest yearnings of the human race can be traced back to this concept of bisexuality. Fantasies of liberation, tragic resignation or reinvention are dominant motives in dreams about the lost self." Perhaps, he wonders, this crime of repression against part of ourselves is the reason why men are essentially afraid of women and vice versa. According to Michael Noll, this dichotomy is represented in the Tarot card, *The Lovers*. The "other" is our twin soul, higher self, and connection to God. Also known as the "dream lovers," this image suggests that the inner being can tell all the secrets of the opposite sex, and how it would feel to be born as the other gender. "You know this person," goes the interpretation, "this person is you" since we all derive from both male and female gametes.

Legends and myths about twins include Esau and Jacob, Romulus and Remus, Castor and Pollox, Leda and the Swan. Perhaps the popularity of these symbols, together with society's fascination with twins, arises from the fact that many more people are unaware of surviving twins that was ever suspected.

Symbols of Implantation

Implantation may be conveyed in feelings of being rooted to the ground, sinking into mud, sand, or a feather bed. The bed is the symbol of the woman, of the mother. Sometimes a devouring animal is the image for threatened uterine resorption by the mother. Drowning, shipwrecks, perishing through exhaustion or being rescued and revived can represent implantation.

Laing linked the following mythical or modern symbols to portray our experience from the stage of a blastula (early ovum development, consisting of a hollow sphere of cells enclosing a cavity) to the epic journey down the tube to the uterus:

BLASTULA

. . . a dome of many-colored glass that stains the white
radiance of eternity

a geodesic dome	a space capsule
a sphere	flying saucer
a balloon	sun-god
the moon	football

the zygote and blastula in the zona pellucida

zona pellucida	first clothing
a box	uterine tube
a casket	the water
an ark	the ocean
a swan	a river

journey along uterine tube to implantation in womb	time in ocean, or drifting down river, till picked up by animals or shepherds, etc.
thus conception uterine journey	in myths birth exposure to sea or river in a box or casket
implantation reception by uterine endometrium	adoption by animals, or lowly people

From R. D. Laing's *The Facts of Life* (New York: Ballantine, 1976).

Symbols of Placenta and Cord

The placenta is the biological center for the regulation of
food and oxygen, and for Mott it was the first instrument of
the unconscious—where we literally have "blood ties." The
fetus projects its own psychic regulation upon the placenta, and

the primitive mind is localized in the placenta in dreams. Femoral arteries (to the legs) are an offshoot from umbilical arteries before birth, so often in myths and dreams there are snakes twisted around legs. Mott also suggested that a sexually indeterminate figure in a dream invariably symbolizes the androgenous placenta. Jung's archetype of the *Shadow* refers to this organ.

HERO	LINKAGE	NURTURING SOURCE
fetus	cord	placenta in womb
	umbilical umbilical	
	arteries vein	
Adam	tree	Eve in garden
	and serpent	
fruit	tree	roots soil
	trunk	
	two-way flow	
	give and take	
St. George	spear	dragon cave
	two snakes	maiden
	staff	
	triple structure	
	caduceus	

From R. D. Laing's *The Facts of Life* (New York: Ballantine, 1976).

Psychotherapist Terence Dowling has also explored placental symbols and the ancient practice of tree therapy. He claims that all mythical stories about trees since the dawn of history represent the "tree of life"—the placenta. We project aspects of our prenatal experience into symbols that, by their shape and configuration, remind us of that experience.

The wicked witch who lives in a tree house conveys the fact that the placenta can be both poisonous and nurturing. The concept of punishment, and some forms of masochism in fantasy and deed, symbolizes the primal condition of the womb, with emphasis on its painful character such as being in chains, feeling intense heat, or being sewn in a sack and sunk in the sea.

The poisonous placenta is often a marine monster (water represents amniotic fluid), even occurring in the myths of lands where there are no snakes. DeMause claims that our "internal punitive agency, the superego, is the fetal image of the poisonous placenta, interfering with the search for love, pleasure and independence."

The umbilical cord is often represented as a flagpole, connecting rope, or snake. The caduceus (the wand of Hippocrates) is the sign of the medical profession and represents the umbilical cord. The mythology of the mysterious serpent on the tree of life and the serpent in the Garden of Eden all draw on the same symbol. The number three features significantly in dreams and legends, representing the three umbilical vessels (three vessels of the cord). Often in myths there are three gates, three bears, three lions, or three dragons, as in Grimms' tale of "The Devil and the Three Golden Hairs." The Scandinavian mythical hero Odin spent nine days (symbolic of pregnancy) on a tree with three roots. The nine guardians at the gates represent the nine months of gestation.

The placenta appears frequently and in various forms: mother's breast, mother's body, excretory pot, eating pot, and the earth. In primitive tribes the placenta was often called the "double," "soul," "secret helper," or "brother," and either was buried or was placed in a tree or on top of a pole.

DeMause's theories include the placental prototype of every god "from whom all blessings flow" and every leader "from whom all power flows." All leaders derive power from being crowned, like a newborn "crowns" at birth, in a rebirth ceremony that confers upon them the "blood power of the worshipped placenta." As Divine Placenta, holder of all placental fetishes—crown, scepter, robe, banner, or flag—the ruler is worshipped as the source of all blood power. In Egypt, the pharaoh led processions preceded by his actual placenta, fixed to the top of a long pole with a dangling umbilical cord. Placental symbols since antiquity have been seen on temples, seals, and shields and in cave paintings. Either treelike or snakelike qualities may be emphasized. The serpent betrays its origin as Poisonous Placenta in every aspect, according to deMause, in "its birth from an egg, in its home in holes or in water, in its role as guardian of the Tree of Life, in its life-giving blood out of which mankind is produced, in its poisonous sting and its ferocious opposition to the mythic hero."

Once the basic pattern becomes familiar, suggested deMause, it is not difficult to see the "elements of the Poisonous Placenta behind *every* malevolent group-fantasy figure in history": sorcerers, menstruating women, blood-poisoning Jews, the red tide of communism. Symbols of the evil placenta abound in political cartoons today. The drama of the suffering fetus, then, is the deepest level of meaning for all rituals, religious or political, in all primitive, archaic, or historical groups, no matter how many elements are present from later life. DeMause explained that:

> once one begins to recognize the limited cast, the standard stage settings, and the ritual script of the fetal drama, what once seemed like endless cultural invention in history and ethnology quickly reduces itself to a few ritual group fantasies endlessly repeated at different evolutionary levels, according to the childrearing modes reached by the group.

DeMause proposed that unless one understands these basic fetal symbols, there is simply no way to explain much of what happens in the world.

Symbols of the Uterus

Visions of fairyland, Atlantis, cities under the sea, treasure hunts, jungle fantasies, historic missions, royal kingdoms, the Garden of Eden, a city of gold, and utopias are based on a biological reality. Conan Doyle's "Lost World" and Rider Haggard's "She" are symbols for the fetal kingdom. The fear and fascination of prenatal return can be seen in legends of the

Lorelei or Tarzan. Apparently, drowning people often curse at lifeguards when they are rescued.

Being in the belly of a ship can indicate pregnancy. The Trojans hid in the belly of a wooden horse. An Egyptian mummy represents mother by name, and symbolically is wrapped the way one's legs or arms were once folded up. The French word la mère (mother) is similar to la mer (sea). A zipper bag is a womb symbol (especially today with so many Cesareans!). Floating and flying are typically uterine memories, as are blindness and darkness.

An item of protection, such as a shield, war chariot, submarine, or tank, at its deepest level signifies a flight to the mother's protective covering. Animal skins in myths and dreams may be a substitute for the protective womb or, as Mott suggested, represent fetal skin; well-known examples include Joseph's coat of many colors and the Golden Fleece, which was nailed to an oak tree and guarded by a sleepless dragon in a sacred grove. Dowling pointed out that the ability to cast off one's skin, like a serpent, is a symbol of rebirth.

We often sleep in the fetal position, and children like to curl up in baskets, boxes, and other small places. Hot tubs, scuba diving, submarines, hot houses, watching plants grow in pots all activate symbolic images of the uterus.

A house may symbolize a woman or a uterus. Rank reminded us of a gruesome ancient custom whereby a living child was walled up in the foundation of a new house, making clear the character of a building as a womb substitute.

A cage, coffin, or dungeon suggests confinement. Fodor pointed out that a "fatalistic touch of resignation in the face of mother's murderous attacks is a typical characteristic of birth dreams . . . birth is the only escape."

Womb imagery is commonly a landscape, a mode of conveyance, or an architectural structure. Thus we see dreams of a garden, park, landscape, or island; a boat, ship, automobile, or railway carriage; a house, room, cellar, basement, loft, cave, or skyscraper. Also symbolic of the uterus is a stove, oven, fireplace, museum, red and blue draperies, church, hotel, raft, or elevator. The "Babes in the Wood" were threatened by a witch that they would be put in an oven.

Water is a frequent image. Boats are universal symbols of the maternal body in which we cross the waters of life: "A symbolic death in water may be the price we have to pay for a new life or rebirth and we are as afraid of paying it now as we were at the time of our first arrival into this world," as Fodor remarked. The sea, lakes, rivers, streams and waterfalls, puddles, tub, toilet, and bathroom are symbols for the amniotic fluid.

Symbols of the Fetus

The fetus, of course, is the mythical hero. He is also represented as the sun, a lion, a king, or other male ruler. The "fetal skin" is represented in dreams as a majestic cloak, a garment of light, or the "mysterious twin." The symbol of the crown goes back to the caul (when the baby is born within intact membranes—a sign of luck). Small animals or insects are symbolic representations of children or embryos, not only on account of their small size but also because of the possibility of their becoming bigger. Eggs, seeds, and plants also represent the fetus, and also worms which grow underground. It is very common for children to form bird's nests with Play-Doh.

LABOR AND BIRTH NIGHTMARES

Nightmare originally referred to an oppressive dream during which the dreamer feels suffocated from pressure on his or her chest, and awakes in fear, gasping for air. Such experiences are said to have originated when the newborn child feels atmospheric pressure on his uninflated lungs and chest. Falling through space or down basement steps or through floorboards that give way are other examples. These nightmares may be recurrent and are usually accompanied by great anxiety, but people wake up before reaching the ground, often around the time of their birth.

Labor typically is described as the feeling of being crushed or compressed, and crawling through a narrow opening. Tunnels, mazes, going down a narrow river on a barge are birth images, but can be as wide-ranging as being in an aggressive crowd to not being able to find where your car is parked.

An experience of running on railroad tracks and being immobilized when the train is coming, or being pursued by Indians or cowboys, is symbolic of labor. The throat is often equated with the vagina and the window is a genital symbol; a front window represents the vagina and a back window symbolizes the anus. There is vaginal symbolism in ravines, cleft rocks. Dreams about teeth, especially falling out, depict birth. It is legendary that tooth extraction may result in an unconscious fantasy of childbirth. In Nancy Cohen's 1991 book *Open Season*, there is such a story, also revealing how state-dependent memory is triggered:

> I was sitting in the dentist's chair and I had been numbed. The dentist had his hands in my mouth, then the assistant was suctioning my saliva. There was a light above me and my heart began to race. I wanted to scream, "Stop!" The only thing being extracted was a tooth—not a baby—and the scars wouldn't show. But I felt as if I was in the operating room all over again and I found myself blinking back tears.

Birth is often symbolized by even more frightening images: drowning; being sucked into a whirlpool, dragged under by sharks or alligators, or strangled by an octopus; being entangled in underbrush or vines; caught in a tornado, fire, storm, earthquake, avalanche, or engulfing lava; and being beaten or paralyzed. Animal images such as being trampled by horses or devoured by wild beasts or monsters also symbolize birth. Burial alive and various forms of slow and painful death at the hands of humans or machinery represent the ordeal of birth. Nightmares of cannibalism; intruding strangers, rapists; murder, torture; phobias of mutilation; fantasies of demonic power; astral projection, reincarnation; crucifixion fantasies; fears of injections; paranoid obsessions; and umbilical fantasies related to incest and homosexuality are other aspects of the symbolic pattern.

A tunnel, cave, arch, bridge, window, or door describes the birth canal. A long passage, stairs, a ladder, slide, crevice, porthole, or manhole (especially next to railway tracks) signifies the vagina. According to Fodor, climbing to heights may be the form in which liberation is expressed by the unconscious mind (the opposite of falling, as in birth). Fear of crowds and close spaces is related to birth. Keeping the window (symbolic gate to life) open is often essential for some people, especially at night. Air hunger may relate to poisoned air or fetal distress.

To cross the brook is a birth symbol for the transition to postpartum life. Bridges may represent the pubic arch, while riverbanks, railroad tracks, and V-shaped structures refer to a mother's legs. Grass, bushes, forest, fur, and hair allude to the pubic region. The hat is another symbol of female genitalia. Passing examinations, as well as being pressed against obstacles, also represents birth.

DeMause observed prenatal symbols during the ritual of circumcision. In the Jewish bris, the moyel gives the infant a yarmulka (placenta) as compensation for his cut-off foreskin and some blood-red wine, exactly as the Australian aborigine gets a bull-roarer (placenta) and some real blood to drink.

Human development is intertwined with transcultural and preexisting systems of symbols and images. As Jung noted, every creative act draws upon the embedded consciousness that is at the root of our humanity. He stressed the vital human need to discover one's internal reality through the cultivation of symbolic life and to live in active, dynamic contact with the collective unconscious and the self. This makes it possible to draw on the enormous resources and wisdom of the ages that lie in the collective psyche.

Accessing Prenatal Events and Preverbal Memories

Those who cannot remember the past are condemned to repeat it.
— GEORGE SANTAYANA

Although ordinary memory may be flawed, Chamberlain reminded us that at a deeper level there is a vastly extended memory, reachable in nonordinary states of consciousness. During a traumatic event, a person is often in shock, and later in normal consciousness is unable to remember very much at all. Yet under hypnosis, crime victims for example, can recall such details as the numbers on a car license plate. The key is to find a bridge between the physiological and verbal levels of experience. The memory is encoded in a state-bound form and thus a person has to get back into a particular state to access the experience. *Regressive association* is the process by which we put two and two together, not by reasoning but by spontaneous feeling.

REPRESSION

Most of us are heavily conditioned to tense our muscles against complete, free expression. We freeze or block sensations and feelings so that we deaden in a certain way or place (or several). Thus, many of us exhibit various degrees of neurosis that serve as a way of coping while keeping pain at bay. We go from one part of the split in our being to the other, but remain in control—in contrast to psychosis, where a person lives in one part of the split only. To cope, we tend to distort, exaggerate, minimize, edit, delete, and use white lies. An upbringing that lacked parental directness and honesty makes it hard for us to feel, for example, when we are angry, hungry, thirsty, tired, need exercise, or feel sexual. As a result, primary impulses to reach out and make contact are repressed in the unconscious with its forbidden drives, and as well by a further layer of character defenses, substitute contacts, and conformist social veneer.

The majority of people undertake a primal journey because of dissatisfaction with their life resulting from "not getting enough" in the womb. They feel cut off from their emotions or shut down in relationships. Problems with motivation and stress are also very common. As Lake noted decades ago, the typical person who is drawn to regressive experience will relate vague complaints such as:

I don't think I have any specific disease, but I feel ill. I just never feel well nowadays. There's nothing in my present life or my actual bodily health to account for the way I feel. I have a definite, but wordless sense of unease, of tension, of something wrong, of something bad going on inside of me. Why should I feel so washed out, so internally weary? I want to ask "What's got into me?"

Rank commented that repression is a means of defense, and an outlet as soon as the individual comes to grief in reality. It is a law of the unconscious mind that one cannot keep pressure locked up indefinitely. Although the original agony is dissociated—pushed away into the unconscious—it is "always retained on reverberating circuits," reemerging in times of stress. Thus, "what alarmed the foetus into defensiveness, surfaces as the defences fail." Inevitable transitions, illness, accidents, divorce and relationship breakdowns, aging, sickness, or shocks provide "an ever-growing opportunity for the pressure to burst forth from the subterranean domains of the mind." The old defenses crumble and the core of the fear that emerges stretches back through the perinatal period, as Lake puts it, "into catastrophic and fearful crises of trust within the intra-uterine environment."

Accessing early memories thus requires finding a way to lift off the lid of repression. There is no one right technique to explore the unconscious mind. Rather, it is a matter of what feels right and how open one is to surrendering to the unknown. This, in turn, depends on one's resources. When the boxed-up feelings, piled high like building blocks, start to tumble down, the beginnings of a new structure need to be in place as a safety net. Clients need supportive relationships wherein they can experience both mutual connections while maintaining healthy boundaries.

CHALLENGES AND CONCERNS

An understandable query about regression concerns safety: "What if someone gets out of hand?" "What if a person's mental or emotional state becomes worse after the experience?" These are legitimate questions. Opening up and letting go can trigger any one of our major fears: (1) the fear of going crazy, (2) the fear of dying, or (3) the fear of either perverse sexual desire or homicidal rage.

Wilhelm Reich pointed out that when there is sufficient emotional charge, buried material will come to the surface, in a safe and supportive environment. If a bodyworker, for example, is apprehensive during a client's emotional response, her or his reticence will be conveyed and the client will shut down. If the facilitator can understand and accept a person's feelings and behavior, then it becomes easier for that person to own and to explore them. In any therapy, the therapist's attitude is a key factor. Optimism about a client's ability to make connections from his or her inner knowing is paramount.

Graham Farrant will not take clients who have had electroshock therapy, who have serious mental health disorders, or who are on medication. (He will also not take smokers, because nicotine is such a barrier to primal experience.)

Stan and Christina Grof do not permit pregnant women to participate in their holotropic breathwork, since the hyperventilation that is encouraged can cause decreased circulation to the placenta. The Grofs have also reported that women will sometimes begin to menstruate in mid-cycle, as a hormonal reaction to the stress.

Most therapists facilitate gentle regression in pregnant women, preferably in the middle trimester, when the baby's embryonic development is complete but the baby is not so large as to make floorwork uncomfortable for the mother. Hypnosis and visualization can be done at any time and have been shown to reduce potential problems with labor and birth, and even reverse complications that may develop such as preterm labor or high blood pressure.

Obviously, common sense is required when going into an altered state of consciousness, like first removing eyeglasses, false teeth, and jewelry. Cathartic floorwork is not suitable for people with seizure disorders, cardiovascular problems such as high blood pressure, or other inappropriate mental or physical health problems.

TECHNIQUES OF ACCESS

The most frequent question asked about reliving early memories is, "How does a person get into that state?" To do is to believe. There are many routes: primal therapy; hypnosis; visualization, holotropic breathwork, rebirthing ("dry"—on land—or "wet"—in a hot tub) aquagenesis: bioenergetics, biosynthesis (grounding, facing, and internal streaming,) orgone or vegetotherapy; energy balancing techniques such as polarity and cranio-sacral therapy—"unwinding"; deep massage such as rolfing; psychoperistaltic massage (in which the therapist listens throughout to intestinal sounds with a stethoscope) meditation; resting in a bath in dark isolation tanks; encounter groups; rites of passage; holding therapy, tribal dancing, shamanic drumming or religious rituals, vision quests; Gestalt or other techniques of humanistic psychology; science fiction or actual space exploration, books and videos showing fetal development, drawing, painting, creating with clay or sand, evocative music, heartbeat sounds, poetry, sex, psychedelic drugs, zero-balancing—the possibilities are unlimited and not listed here in any rank order. For a woman, giving birth is a potentially powerful regression experience, just as reliving being born can be mixed with a woman's own experiences of labor and delivery.

Unintentional regression can occur during viral illnesses such as flu, infection, and hepatitis. Fevers, hyperthyroidism, goiter, premenstrual syndrome, prolonged sleep or food deprivation, motion sickness, and sea sickness all diminish the forces of repression. Drugs that abolish consciousness, anesthetics, barbiturates, and alcohol also weaken repression, either when they take effect or when their effect is wearing off.

With infants and children, California psychotherapist William Emerson uses large womb sheets—twenty by twenty-five feet. Together with heart beat rhythms, sand play, and a large range of figures, animals, and symbolic representations, Emerson easily assists regression in his small patients. He has found that 30 percent of sand play is prebirth—choosing an embryo, fetus, making womb structures, and using sperm and egg symbols that indicate conception. Emerson has worked extensively with conception trauma in infants. While the parents talk about conception, he watches the reaction of the infant, and in about 10 to 15 percent of cases, the babies respond with crying that indicates trauma. Emerson then asks the parents to elaborate further. Colic, breastfeeding difficulty, and projectile vomiting are some of the problems Emerson sees with an unplanned conception.

Psychotherapist Terence Dowling uses a simple diagnostic game with a six-foot-long dark tunnel made of soft material. He treats groups or individual children after the age of about eighteen months. Clues to pre- and perinatal experience can be observed in the way children relate to and move through the tunnel. One child who had been ambivalent at first could actually tolerate very strong blocking of the exit without any signs of panic. He pushed and shouted and never became passive. Suddenly he crashed through the *side* of the tunnel and ran to his mother. She reported that he was an emergency Cesarean birth.

Music can be a powerful facilitator of emotion and memory, and Stan Grof details a wonderful collection of music for regression in *The Adventure of Self-Discovery*. On the other hand, silence has a place, too.

I have tried many of the approaches listed above, and most have presented me with different glimpses into my primal reality. Isolated in a flotation tank, for example, I felt for the first time the tension in my eye muscles, anchored in tight neck muscles. (There are connections with the autonomic nervous system—our fight-flight-fright reactions—through the blood supply to the eyes.) Marijuana brought up my issues with time, with a few minutes seeming like hours. Polarity therapy helped me to sense the split between my left and right sides and a block in my left shoulder blade. Rebirthing and holotropic breathing does not work for me because one of my primal issues was the decision to be alive and to breathe. The requirement to breathe in a specific way interferes with my core experience of not breathing. In my experiences of both hypnosis and rebirthing, I felt too much direction from the facilitator. Some people are comfortable with hypnosis because it does not seek to bring about abreaction, in contrast to the expressive body therapies, which are certainly undignified. Hypnosis fascinates me, but I prefer sound, movement, and the opportunity to let go of words. A large part of language is nonverbal; body language is the way children communicate before they learn to speak. Likewise, with age regression it can be important to relive the nonverbal experiences through the body initially, letting words come later.

I believe that resonance is the catalyst for any activity between the client and the facilitator; the method is secondary. Primarily, there must a commitment to feel one's truth at the deepest level, especially when others—with the best of intentions—help the client avoid feeling inner pain. It takes a lot of courage to risk being as honest as the regression process demands and to search for the truth with heart and soul. I have also found that clients will present me with a "trivial" symptom as a way of investigating me, to check if they feel safe enough to let out the real issue. Reassurance that "things are not so bad" or "could have been worse" is counterproductive because it undermines the client's personal reality. Instead I affirm and encourage the expression of their feelings, particularly the negative emotions.

Visualization

Visualization and guided fantasy are probably the most popular techniques for getting into a moderately altered state of consciousness. These approaches can be done with individuals or groups and with people sitting in chairs. Most people in the West are predominantly visual, but auditory and kinesthetic aspects are of prime importance for some individuals as are suggestions of taste and smell, and the use of music and other sound effects enhances the suggestions, as does synesthesia (providing an experiential quality by appropriate voice modulation to something high, low, soft, etc.).

I have created a guided visualization for exploring inside experiences from conception through birth; see Appendix 1. This forty-five-minute experience has been well received by my groups for over a decade. Most people have some recall of pre- and perinatal events, and not infrequently a vivid breakthrough and connection. An audiocassette tape of the guided visualization with specially composed music is also available in several languages; see the Resources section.

Body-Oriented Therapies

I prefer to work with an individual client on the floor in a small, safe room. My original training was in physical therapy, an invaluable foundation of involving touch and movement and a thorough understanding of the body. Generally, clients consult me for a somatic condition, which may or may not have pre- and perinatal origins. This is a distinction that I arrive at through my intuition, the client's body language and his or her use of metaphors. I also take a detailed history and genogram as in Appendix 2. My multi-faceted approach mobilizes the client's potential for health. I may do manual adjustments, stretches, exercises, biofeedback and so on, plus guided regression. Clients more often than not prefer (and I give them the choice) to spend more time on the couch or the floor, as they go deeper into understanding their body-mind interactions, knowing that I support every dimension of their personal reality without judging or reassuring. This is very *physical* therapy!

In my present location, I have a safe soundproofed room, away from distractions. This symbolic uterus has padded foam on the floors and walls, covered with red fake fur. The dimmable lights are red, too. Here I have the options of many approaches: to make contact or just be a presence; to use music, sound, hypnosis, visualization, affirming comments or remain silent; to facilitate and provoke, or to contain and calm the client (especially if a child or baby).

Boadella pointed out that going from lying down to standing up can be compared with our evolution from water to land, which is also the developmental achievement of the human being during gestation. Alexander Lowen, founder with John Pierrakos of Bioenergetics, stressed "grounding exercises" in standing—learning to fall and be caught—and opening the chest cavity by lying backward over a breathing stool. It is always important to experience the *process*—for example, transitions between positions—without being orientated to a goal or end-product.

A person's inner desire to interact with his or her surroundings may be inhibited by shame, guilt, panic, or defeat. Whatever the cause, personal resources are not translated into movement. Marcher and Jarlness have designed a system called "body mapping," in which they note the degree of tone in all the muscles, marking them with different colors on a diagram. The cause of insufficient tone in a muscle is a lost impulse, a giving up before a movement was even begun. In contrast, tense muscles result when the movement was initiated but then suddenly suppressed. Certain muscles become active at specific phases of development, therefore variations in muscle tone provide a map of a person's preverbal being.

Groups can be used to simulate pressure of the uterus and birth canal and to provide rocking experiences. For example, three people can form a unit with the middle one being the fetus, and perform flexion and extension movements to represent contraction and relaxation of the uterus.

Lisbeth Marcher points out that during birth, contractions force the baby into smaller space until he actively begins to push against it. He senses his own power in the stretch reflex, extending against the pressure of the uterus as actively as a chicken pecks its way out of the egg. People with healthy births can honor their own power: "They are confident that they can tolerate pressure and stress, can be active and self-directed and still be welcomed and loved." That synthesis has to be recreated in therapy by finding new physical, mental and emotional resources.

Integrated Respiration Therapy and Haptonomy (the science of touch and feeling) are primarily existential philosophies but the experience of deep contact facilitates recall of early memories. I have personally experienced Frans Veldman's haptonomic approach. This charismatic man skillfully reduces a person's abdominal skin reflexes and involuntary muscle tone within minutes. Haptonomy is widely practiced in Europe as psychotherapy (reaffirming the inherent good in each person, reestablishing his or her felt base of security) as well as prenatal preparation (ideally commencing before conception).

The central concept of Integrated Respiration Therapy is that a person is whole and needs only to be awakened. Lillemor Johnsen does not concentrate on tense muscles; in fact, she respectfully avoids a defense and trusts that it will leave when it is not needed. Defenses help the patient to keep functioning and if not respected, the original symptom is replaced by another and may shift from the muscles to the viscera. Rather than working through the pathological, she helps to release the "repressed psychic material and expressive potential" from underdeveloped lax muscles. Her hand is the instrument of discovery, with "ear-fingertip listening" to encourage the latent content to breathe and live again. There are no exercises, manipulations, or breath training: it is a silent interaction.

Johnsen's aim is both to liberate respiration—to experience it throughout the whole body—and to draw earlier nonintegrated experiences back into the personality. The tools here are free associations, bodily expression, and dream material. The muscles are integrated with the respiration at the exact moment when the psychic contents are integrated in the personality:

> The respiratory capacity points to an expressive capacity, something held back but moveable. When respiration is complete, streaming, harmonious and spontaneous, it is integrated in one's musculature, personality and speech. When integration takes place, when muscles live again, memory also lives.

Veldman has different charts that show the variation in respiration: for example, listening to different kinds of music or an argument, or being in real contact with another person (when the rhythms synchronize). Boadella contrasts blocked fear as a reluctance to breathe in; with blocked anger, a reluctance to breathe out.

Psychedelics

Psychedelics are rarely used to access prenatal experiences because of medical, legal, and political restrictions. However, their use has been culturally widespread and they are undoubtedly effective in opening the "doors of perception," as Aldous Huxley wrote in one of the first books on this subject. Historically, these substances have played an important role in forcing a paradigm shift to understand better the realms of the human unconscious.

Like Grof, Lake used LSD extensively with patients and found that at least half of them relived, reenacted, and described their "transition through the birth passages." Although not all of the birth experiences were painful, Lake observed "severe crushing as well as mental pain beyond the limits of tolerance." Indeed, he was not prepared for the frequent abreaction of birth trauma and the re-living of specific birth injuries such as forceps delivery, the cord around the neck, and various other dramatic episodes that were

> so vivid, so unmistakable in their origin, and afterward confirmed by the mother or other reliable informants that my scepticism was shaken. Nothing would convince the patient that this was a fantasy. Various positions of head and body as they rotated in second stage of labour are reproduced as if by the same irresistible external force. Trapped limbs again feel trapped and crushed. Motor, sensory nerves and the autonomic nervous system are all activated.

Lake stated that without exception those who had undergone both mystical experiences or traumatic depersonalization were "confident that they belong, without any question, to the earliest months of their life." The first category contained the positive feelings of a preverbal, pretransition union with the mother in the "womb of the spirit" and the second contained the pain of an "unsupportable fission" from her.

Hypnosis

Hypnosis was used during surgery before the development of anesthetic agents; it offered the *only* relief in those days. Like acupuncture, it has a high success rate, especially when there are no alternatives. Hypnosis has been effective during birth for patients who are motivated, but the popularity of anesthesia and medication nowadays has decreased people's incentive to go the drugless route. Hypnotism and hypnotherapy, unfortunately, have sometimes suffered from a bad press ranging from theatrical associations to domineering practitioners to accusations about the power of suggestion. However, just because suggestion is an aid to memory retrieval does not mean that the primal memories are a result of suggestion. In keeping with humanistic psychotherapies today, the goal is not to find the "right answer," but rather to activate inner processes and resources in the client. Then connections and healing happen without much input from the therapist, and in fact often occur spontaneously.

People enter a light hypnotic state when they are in the process of remembering any sequence of events. Formal induction of hypnosis such as counting backward or watching the flame of an imaginary candle is not always necessary. Cheek outlined two methods for questioning subjects under hypnosis. One is to use a pendulum on a chain that may swing in three directions predetermined by the client, representing "Yes," "No," and "I don't want to answer" (or "I am not willing to talk about that yet"). The other technique was to use prearranged finger signals for those three answers. It is important that memories be re-experienced at physiological and ideomotor (finger or pendulum movements) levels, sometimes even many times, *before* being verbalized. The pendulum or the finger signals are more accurate than any verbal statements, because unconscious body movements are more reliable than conscious recall. Often the most significant ideomotor signals are barely visible but convincingly repetitive.

Individuals understandably resist the recall of painful events. Cheek described two approaches that he uses. One is to go over the experience as it might have been, if all the right things had been done and the memories were pleasant. The second approach is to go back before the event occurred. The first is more cathartic emotionally, whereas the retrospective approach is more effective in desensitizing traumatic memories.

It may be necessary to keep going around the experience, rephrasing and reframing it, to get past unconscious resistance. The client is asked to go back earlier and earlier to the original trauma. He or she may be asked if the answer given is the whole answer, and if it is all right to tell the hypnotherapist about it. Subjects can be guided back and forth out of hypnosis to find out with which levels of memory they are comfortable. Clients can be given the option of the present or past tense, and of saying "I'm not ready to know the answer consciously *yet,*" to postpone further delving to a later time. *Yet* implies that understanding *will* come; this optimistic expectation is affirming for the client. Likewise, Cheek will sometimes say, "Let your inner mind give a yes signal when it is ready to pop the date of a completely satisfactory resolution of that problem into your conscious mind." Then he will close by stating that the client has experienced enough of a stressful situation for now, and guide the individual to return to normal consciousness, alert and refreshed.

Reframing and rescripting help the client to reinterpret and re-structure events with adult perception. He can imagine ideal situations or something deeply desired, to transform his sense of deprivation. With updated resources, perhaps including spiritual insights, the energy that lay beneath the constraints and limitations can be released. Affirmations can assist the metamorphosis.

Physician Lewis Mehl found that 75 of 100 patients who came to him for hypnosis to help resolve physical symptoms experienced prenatal memories. Seventeen relived the onset of their current problem as during the prenatal phase of their lives. These patients were shocked to remember that their mothers did not want them or even wished to abort them. The mothers were sad, depressed, and frustrated by the pregnancy and the fathers were enraged at the news, often for financial reasons.

Mehl describes the case of Terri, who while still inside her mother remembered the traumatic suicide of an aunt. The family had decided to conceal the suicide because they were Catholic, and were amazed that Terri knew because she had been a fetus of only ten weeks at the time. The ramifications of this family pattern of concealment had important consequences for Terri's physical problems and their amelioration.

Primal Therapy

Primal therapy was originated by psychologist Arthur Janov in the early seventies. Since that time, the process has been modified by different practitioners around the world. Primaling involves floorwork with encouragement to move, make sound, and abreact on all levels, as case histories throughout the book illustrate.

Clients have expressed their preferences as follows:

I've tried psychedelic drugs, but they just bypass the situation. . . . I couldn't do yoga because of the pain, until I did primal therapy, then I could let out the pain. This gave me a sense of emotional and physical relief and connectedness with every cell in my body.

I just wonder how conventional therapies work. For me, it takes more energy now to resist than release. I feel as if I have no space to move, and if anything goes wrong I think it is my fault. I allow the feeling to come up without judging, analysis, criticism, interpretation, and cure. I slow down my thoughts and become very aware, and trust my movements. . . . They become the core, the essence of an evolving knowing of what I want to do, to move, to express, and feel.

There is a dramatic shift into body awareness. Today I stood up, symbolically growing up. I stood tall, felt stronger, assertive, all body directed. Although it felt different, it's me and I know the challenge is to continue that in the outside world.

One advantage of primal work is the future independence. (Self-hypnosis can also be learned and audiotapes can be purchased for guided visualization.) As a client's trust and ability to let out buried terror and rage increase, he or she gains the courage to be alone and to experience spontaneous outpourings, without needing a facilitator or any special equipment. As one person described the process:

You just lie down, close eyes, and relax. If you lie long enough, the mind searches for distractions, you fidget. Sometimes I talk out loud and get into it, or I focus on a part of myself, or on the area of my body that is fidgeting. Thereafter no more is required as the body's memories take over and you do what you have to do.

Positive Primal Experiences

People describe embryonic, oceanic bliss quite commonly. This merging, melting, harmonic unity is linked to the development of spiritual feelings. It is not uncommon for individuals to describe conception as an experience of trinity: sperm, egg, and Holy Ghost or cosmic life force.

Experiences of bliss, God, a higher power, cosmic force, life energy, and universal love usually occur in the period before fertilization through to early uterine existence. (This is the period before most mothers are conscious of the pregnancy.) Such transpersonal and spiritual feelings are felt as much stronger and larger than oneself. One woman said:

Enclosed in the uterus, I experienced sensual feelings of intense love, that I could touch, and give out. I loved being in the womb. I can now see the love around me in my partner. I got born in one big step when I finally made up my mind. Then after doing it, I was crying with the abandonment.

Hanspeter Ruch is a twin and clinical psychologist in Winterthur, Switzerland. As part of his academic research he underwent primal therapy to journey back to his life in the womb. Ruch wrote in his master's thesis:

My early life in utero, in paradise was like:
swimming in the warm ocean
floating and flying
being cuddled in a waterbed
being massaged by gentle waves
being a stream of warmth and sunshine
being harmony, happiness, joy
being a unity
being freedom and beauty
being peacefulness, safety, comfort
being lightness, softness, gentleness and
weightlessness
just being—no words.

There are usually positive moments even in the most troubled beginnings. Some peaceful and warm memories are mentioned in unhappy anecdotes but in general, pain predominates in our imperfect world.

THE USE OF LANGUAGE

Language is often used as a defense against feelings rather than to focus them. It is difficult to feel deeply while talking. In my group work with touch experiences, I always request silence until the end of the interactions. Paul Tournier put it very well in his *The Meaning of Persons*:

> The language of the human heart, when it casts off the intellectualism in which it has been trained at school and recovers its pristine freshness . . . is the language of our dreams. The thing that strikes me when I am talking with my patients is that the moment deep personal contact is made, the very style of our talk changes. Images spring spontaneously to the mind, we begin to talk in parables, and we understand one another better than when the tone of the conversation was intellectual and didactic. The conversation becomes anecdotal, as the Bible is anecdotal, as the *Iliad* and the *Odyssey* are anecdotal, but the anecdote is no longer then merely a story, it is an experience, a personal truth.

Johnsen emphasizes the importance of spontaneous rhymes, songs and jingles, joy, creativity, and childish expression. Her books contain many examples of unusual sentence construction, imagery, and word play.

FACETS OF FACILITATION

An individual needs first to believe that regression is possible and therapeutic, and to feel ready and committed. Even then, most people find it difficult, initially, to let go. Our defenses serve us thoroughly and take time to be dismantled. We intuitively protect ourselves from going too far too soon. And coercion is not possible, since the process is one of softening and surrender.

Anxiety can arise simply when an individual lies on his or her back, with arms and legs uncrossed, in a darkened room. Therefore, it is helpful if novices are given a thorough introduction to the dimensions of regression by people who have happily survived the experience, using videotapes that show the potential range of emotional expression and abreaction.

Accessing labor and birth experiences takes longer for people whose mothers were given drugs and anesthesia—a common experience. During regression, these people may go limp, black out, smell ether, become numb, or feel in a fog. One woman always felt that when her mother came into the room she was taking her air and became breathless. An anesthesiologist felt so suffocated in a primal room that she brought in equipment to measure the percentage of oxygen in the air! (Subsequently, she experienced the anesthetic given to her mother at birth and connected it with her choice of medical specialty.)

Conscious resistance (typically experienced as anxiety) and unconscious defenses are obstacles to accessing inner experiences. Do we enter the world in the "fight" mode or in the "passive death" mode? asks Janov. Analysis and intellectualization also stand in the way and often serve as defenses for articulate people. Some people hang on to their pain tenaciously, because letting go of it means facing the unknown, an agonizing void, the "dread of nothingness." On the other hand, there are some individuals who readily get into explosive discharges or hysterics, or act out; for them it is a challenge to contain themselves and their breathing as they stay with a feeling. Regression itself can be a defense.

Janov observed that when sensations are persistent in a patient, "we know the Pain is near—constant coughing, a continual lump in the throat, a tautness in the neck and shoulders." Breaking through these sensations is known as *first-line intrusion*. This comes from first-line primal pressure, indeed a physiological pressure that can be measured. The earlier the pain, the higher the blood pressure; it can mount to well over 200 mmHg. Likewise, there are significant changes in brain-wave patterns and in the electrical output of muscle groups.

FEELING SAFE

The more a person can let his inner self be seen by another, the more recognizable he becomes to himself. Real depth of self-exposure is possible only in the presence of a trusted person. The term *therapist* comes from the Greek *therapoien*, meaning "someone who accompanies." A person who has confronted his or her inner demons helps others feel safe to do the same. Whether they have a Ph.D. or M.D. or not, the therapist's integrity is validated by his or her own courage in having made the journey personally, and the individual can remain calm and secure, knowing that while clients may *feel* they are stifled, strangled, have to vomit, and so on, these are "just" feelings —a personal reality but not actual events in the present.

Intuition, which develops with experience, is also necessary since this phenomenological process is unpredictable. A facilitator must be completely open, fearless, warm, and compassionate to encourage a full expression of whatever feeling state has emerged.

Another important attribute is a sense of trust that the path is the *process*, with no goals or judgments in mind. Like birth, the client has to lose control, to get out of his or her head to get into his or her body—a total surrender. In the beginning, it is extremely frightening to go back to a state of total powerlessness and vulnerability. One has to let go of all goals, plans, expectations, and frameworks and leap into the unknown. This is emotionally risky and terrifying. So often a person will say, "I'm afraid to cry for what will all come out," or "Once I start, I'll never be able to stop." On the other hand, a person's "empty core" may be devastating. But as philosopher Alan Watts said, "let yourself be afraid and then you can release the fear."

Ideally, discharge begins gently, until it is integrated with consciousness. In reliving early events, clients must have the freedom to do it their way. As in a birth, they need enough time, must learn to tolerate pressure and take an active role.

A network of supporting relationships helps the client find the strength to live through overwhelming primal memories.

Empathy, affirmative sounds and words, gentle suggestions, physical assistance or resistance, massage, and pressure on a key area like the head, chest, feet, or umbilicus can help the process. Abreaction involves discharge from the autonomic nervous system—tears, gagging, bringing up mucus, sobbing, trembling, involuntary muscle spasms, and attaining postures and performing movements that are difficult or impossible voluntarily. The odor of fear in primal groups is quite remarkable; likewise, it was the smell of fear that Romans masked when they covered their body with scented oil before a battle.

Catharsis is physiological as well as emotional. Emotions are always expressed in the body; the word *emotion* comes from the Latin *emovere*—to move away and, as D. H. Lawrence put it poetically:

The body's life is the life of sensations and emotions. The body feels real hunger, real thirst, real joy in the sun or the snow, real pleasure in the smell of roses or the look of a lilac bush, real anger, real sorrow, real tenderness, real warmth, real passion, real hate, real grief. All the emotions belong in the body and are only recognized by the mind.

During even the most explosive catharsis one is always aware of a part of the self that is like a detached observer, but at the same time is central and fundamental. This is the part that knows that "the only way out is all the way in."

The word *try* has no place in this process because it creates performance anxiety, effort, and body tension. The permissive mode is essential: to allow . . . experience . . . let yourself go back . . . trust your body to express. In order to disengage the intellect, it's helpful to let words fall away; let your body express the feeling, thought, or emotion.

Likewise, "I don't know" is not acceptable, and in hypnosis, there is no finger signal for that phrase; instead you must admit that you do know, but don't want to answer. It is often the case that a *part* of yourself knows, feels, can move, or can express some emotion. You can stay deeply with the present or entertain the opposite idea. How would it be if you *didn't* hit, hold your breath, or lie still, for example?

Feeling inner pain is generally followed by new and rewarding feelings: agony and relief are opposite sides of the same experience. Therapeutic re-enactment helps us to withdraw projections from the past. One person admitted that "actual physical pain can feel okay because it feels right, real. I need to finalize a primal feeling and get it out of my system." It is like a rebirth, as there can be positive pain in birth, pain *without suffering*.

Pain usually arises from resistance, and when the resistance is released, new energy flows forth, characteristically in breath and sound. The voice expresses or blocks vibrations from the body's core and the voice quality changes as a person begins to loosen the chains of repression. People make all kinds of sounds—moans, cries, chants, grunts, screams, jibberish, baby talk. (A scream is a tool, not the therapy!) Occasionally clients will even speak in a foreign language that they heard only as an unborn baby. Unconscious material may be relived in dramatic forms involving birth, death, and transpersonal phenomena (including past lives, experiences from other cultures and languages, even identification with other species) as Grof described in *Realms of the Human Unconscious*.

It is vital to contact good feelings while discharging bad ones. Often one will realize, for example, that a *part* of mother's psyche wanted the pregnancy or that her anxiety was not a result of the pregnancy but rather an external situation. The pain of denied needs forces the heart aside, so that it is protected in a deep place where it may even be forgotten. One of the rewards of making an inner journey is the glimpse of a state of grace and the joyful awakening to one's heartfelt center.

Primal Group Experiences

Group experiences offer different dynamics, a shared higher energy, "permission" by others in a similar state to experience—and to voice—one's truths. Getting in touch with issues about personal space, and the opportunity to learn how to express feelings in an upright position and to other people, is also significant, as this client expressed:

> In one group, I stretched out and bumped one of the sitters. Naturally I recoiled my foot, but she took it and straightened it beside her. The most overwhelming feeling of being wanted, or having a right to that space, came over me and quiet tears rolled.
>
> Later I was back to feeling angry and repressed and yet someone else was there pushing hard on my head, stopping me from moving. I felt I had to get out or else I'd die, and this became more and more desperate. I did push through and I felt that unless I could express my feelings I would die. And the only way I could do this was to be big. When I finally opened my eyes I was standing against the wall across the room from where I'd begun. I don't remember getting there, but though exhausted, I felt strong. It was also the first time I'd been upright in the group. Soon after I remembered my mother saying that my birth was rapid, too quick for the doctor to get there and the nurses had tried to hold me back.

Before I began my inner journey, I was not looking for any of the approaches I have just described. For me, it was a case of being in the right place at the right time after my labor experience had defied rational understanding. A series of events led me to Graham who helped me to solve the riddles of my early existence and to enjoy greater authenticity in my present life.

A Turning Point: My Inner Journey Begins

*When I remember an incident in my life, I can recall it two ways,
from "inside" or "outside" as it were.*

—R. D. LAING

My first experience with regression was in 1982, when I spent several days studying bioenergetics with Eva Reich, M.D., the daughter of Wilhelm Reich, whose psychological insights I had admired for a long time. Bioenergetics incorporates regression as it encourages the free flow of the body's energy and concomitant emotional release. The process began for me when I was surrounded by several people who formed a "uterus" around me with pillows. Rather than immediately fighting to get free of the pressure (as commonly happens), I simply decided not to breathe. Eva became so alarmed at this response that she terminated the experience, saying "You were a SIDS baby in utero—I don't want to work with you again unless I have oxygen available." The rest of the group commented with amazement that I had looked just like a fetus during the experience.

Having been born at home without any complications, I never felt drawn to relive my birth. I was thus surprised and confused by my unhappy feelings in the "uterus" that day. I hadn't contemplated issues from time *before* birth. So I just set them aside and turned my interest toward watching the skill and compassion with which Eva led people into their deeper feelings over the next few days.

My Meeting with Graham Farrant

I am often surprised about the timing of events, which makes our universe seem less random and more benevolent. Sometimes I buy a book that sits on my bookshelf for months or years. One such title was Arthur Janov's *The Primal Scream*, which in 1982 I decided to take along on a trip to the Orient and South Pacific, and was soon engrossed.

I had read most of the book when I met the physical therapist in Sydney who had suffered the car accident which she subsequently related to her birth, as I described in the Introduction. I was looking forward to meeting her psychiatrist Graham Farrant, but I didn't anticipate an initiation into an altered state of consciousness.

I drove with my husband Geoff and eight-month-old Julia down Erin Street, in an inner suburb of Melbourne, lined with turn-of-the-century terrace houses, most of them converted to medical offices. As we searched for number 57, Graham appeared in the street right before our car. With uncanny timing he had stepped out to greet us. I knew from the clarity of his eyes that he was the "primal man."

We were ushered into his office in the front of the townhouse and introduced to several of his staff. Then Graham asked me, "What do you know about your birth?" "Oh," I replied, "I was born at home, and as the story goes, in one contraction." I was not prepared for unanimous laughter that followed. This mirth arose from the fact that Graham, after one of my hasty phone calls from Sydney, had announced to the staff in his office that a woman from the United States was coming to visit who "sounded like she had been born in one contraction!"

As an obstetric physical therapist and childbirth educator, I had never really understood how a baby could be born in just one or even a few contractions. Were there really so few contractions, or did a woman such as my mother simply not perceive them? Certainly in such a birth it is a strong "fetal ejection reflex"—not much labor is required on the mother's part! I had listened to the story of my birth ad nauseam, especially from my father. Since my parents had not planned a home birth, they were caught quite unprepared and coped without any medical assistance.

I was deeply struck by Graham's intuition. How could he sense a person's birth history from a couple of phone calls? I also had the unanswered questions about Julia's birth. When Graham volunteered that professionals in the birth field were attracted to their occupation because of their own primal experiences, I felt that I was on the edge of a huge precipice. I also knew I had no choice but to jump, terrifying as it was, because it felt right.

On Graham's suggestion, I returned the next day by myself to experience a group music session. I entered the large red room at the back of the house and lay down with my towel in an unoccupied corner. A red light shone dimly on the walls and floor, which were covered with red silk. Underneath, thick foam padded every surface. Bodies were scattered on the floor in various degrees of disarray. I stole looks and listened nervously. Some people lay deathly still; others twitched and jerked, groaned and moaned, occasionally moving into a crescendo of catharsis. If I hadn't read *The Primal Scream* and learned about the extremes of emotional expression, I might have panicked and fled. Nevertheless, my heart was pounding. I didn't know what I was supposed to do, what would happen, what the ground rules were.

The music was transporting and ranged from classical to African drums to Gregorian chants to melancholy pop. I lay down for what seemed a long time, feeling doleful and apprehensive. Soon my bladder felt as if it would burst. I left the room and headed for the toilet, only to be grabbed by one of the staff who sternly dictated: "You may not leave the group and you may not use the bathroom."

I felt both enraged and terrified. I'd noticed the door opening and closing as other people came and left. Who was this bitch to tell me I couldn't leave to pee? Why weren't these crazy rules explained first? Resentfully, I lay down again with my bladder at the point of explosion and prayed for it all to be over.

Soon I became aware of someone sitting beside me. From

under my half-closed lids I saw it was Graham. He gently laid his hand on the top of my chest and said, "What are you feeling?" Sadness welled up and I struggled to explain it. "You don't have to be clever," he said, "Just be *you*." As I stayed with the sadness, I recognized that it was a very familiar feeling. As I let myself go back to the first time I had felt that way, I knew that it was from my life inside my mother. I was surrounded by an all-pervasive state of grief that I did not understand. The feeling of grief competed with the bursting pressure in my bladder and I shifted from one painful state to the other.

Mercifully the music came to an end, the lights were turned up, and people slowly roused themselves to a sitting position. The floor was littered with tissues, and everyone looked wrung out. After enough time passed for people to dry their eyes and orient themselves, Graham asked who wanted to share. I felt like the new kid on the block and fervently hoped I wouldn't have to say a word. Actually, my own feelings diminished as I listened to myriad varieties of primal pain expressed by the group. The sounds of choking, gagging, struggling, kicking, I learned, were all connected to mothers who wouldn't push, babies who couldn't breathe, doctors who pulled and cut, and so on, resulting in feelings of rage, terror, helplessness, distrust, and grief. I was astounded that Graham's insights were not confined to the birth experience but included early pregnancy, implantation, and even back to conception.

Again, I was both fearful and fascinated by the thought of regressing to a stage of such vulnerability. All the criticisms indelibly stamped in my memory from my childhood flooded back to me. Who would want to go back into the deepest levels of old hurts?

I did want to know if *I* could relive my birth and the months before, now that I was reasonably convinced that others certainly had. My curiosity was both professional and personal; I had a strong intuition that work on myself would help to develop and enrich my work with patients. I decided to take the plunge, and planned to return to Graham's clinic in a year for an "intensive." Since I was not seeking therapy, I would not have undergone the process with anyone else. I was reassured by the fact that Graham was a medical doctor, with graduate psychiatric degrees from Harvard and McGill universities. Plus, he had years of experience and also primaled regularly himself. I admired his courage to commit himself to an unorthodox form of psychiatry that he enriched with his own style and spirituality.

THE JOURNEY CONTINUES

An intensive at Graham's clinic takes one to three weeks, during which time the client lives at the clinic, which has a bedroom, bathroom, and kitchen. A faster breakdown of defenses occurs when a person is isolated from outside influences, which enables the process to be experienced as deeply and fruitfully as possible. Regression is exhausting and it is necessary to rest and sleep between sessions, and generally to sink fully into the process without any outside distractions.

I was scheduled for just a one-week residential intensive rather than three because I was coming for curiosity, not psychiatric reasons. During the first week I spent five hours each day in either individual or group sessions. For the second week of my intensive I stayed with friends but visited Graham's office all day, and during the third week, I tapered off in preparation for my return to the United States. (Clients at the clinic typically continue with group and individual sessions for several months after completing an intensive. They have their own key and can use the primal room at any time.)

The intensive began when Graham arrived to get me started with three drawings. I had to sketch myself, him, and a scene. I thought I had achieved a reasonable rendering of my naked self, not knowing that rarely does anyone do the self-portrait without clothing! This, I learned later, alerted Graham that I was making a definitive statement about my female gender!

My scene was a sketch of the pond where I lived on Cape

Cod. This reflected my desire to live by water. Although I grew up in Australia and looked at the horizon of an ocean, I prefer the perimetry of a lake, a primal feeling to do with borders and zones about which I would learn more as I underwent the process and understood my use of prenatal symbols.

BACK TO THE UTERUS

During my first private session with Graham, I lay in semi-darkness on the red silk-covered foam, experiencing cold feet, literally and metaphorically. Graham was astute in noticing any twitch or tremor and gently directed my awareness to that part of my body, with various affirmative sounds and words. He helped intensify what was naturally happening, asking if it was a familiar sensation or feeling, and offering encouragement to go back to earliest time when that same feeling or sensation occurred. Instead of directing my breathing, Graham drew attention to its quality with suggestions such as, "Notice how it feels to hold your breath" or "How would it feel if you didn't hold your breath?"

Somehow we began to discuss my school, which I hated, and the school uniform, which I loathed. From there I moved into deeper feelings of sadness, which I described to Graham, of feeling "not right"—wrong gender, wrong parents, wrong house, wrong school, wrong country. And, Graham pointed out, my first house was my mother's uterus.

As I lay in the dark red glow of the little padded room, he asked me to become aware of how I felt in that first house. My rational mind had already validated his insight; I felt "wrong." I started to cry, to feel wretched. I was most reluctant to stay with these unpleasant feelings. He gently encouraged with such empathy, such "knowing" sounds ("Mmmm. . . . Y-e-s," etc.) that I dared to go a little with the feelings. I noticed that they would build and fade, and there would be a little break between. Each time, however, the wave of feeling would gain a little more momentum, and my body would respond more spontaneously. I felt as if my conscious thoughts, while never absent, were moving into the background and my body was the more powerful and natural vehicle of expression.

The "wrong" feeling was familiar, but I was not prepared for the intense grief that came up. A blanketing feeling of sadness came on, as I had briefly experienced with Eva Reich and the introductory group session at Graham's clinic. *Why all this grief?* What had *I* done to deserve this? I alternated between feeling wronged and angry, and then sad and desolate. The worst part was the deathly stillness I sensed. "Yes, that was it—death; something, someone died." "*I don't want to feel this.*" "I don't want to stay inside, but I don't want to come out." Outside, I sensed, was disappointment and anger. "No place feels right, no place feels that it is for me." "What did all this mean?" I could identify the feelings—indeed, I lived them profoundly—but not yet their context.

During one session I came to understand my immobilization during my labor with Julia, and my inability to void. My bladder was a key area for me and, I have since learned, for many other women. It is for good reason that we have the phrase in English, to be "pissed off" at someone. Women often displace their anger and their tears into their bladders, which plays a role in the common complaint of urinary stress, incontinence, and other bladder dysfunction.

In several previous sessions, feelings of a bursting bladder would come on immediately, it seemed, when I lay down on the floor, even if just minutes before I had just voided. I reluctantly trusted Graham when he said that there was an emotion involved that I had to confront. During one session I just knew I couldn't hold the pissed-off feelings in any longer, but how humiliating if I peed on the red silk floor, and in a group session! I couldn't imagine that the feelings could come out in any other way. Graham *insisted* that I stay with the pain, and said he would get me a plastic sheet. A century of excruciating agony seemed to pass (a deliberate delay) before he returned with the plastic.

I began to understand how women could ask for an epidural in labor—my bladder pain was unbearable. I had to remain on my back to stay with my bladder pain, and it seemed physiologically impossible to void in that position, which also increased the pain. I was completely terrified and the agony was so intense that I lost all sense of observing or feeling that pain—I was the pain and the pain was me.

Graham encouraged me to let the pain have a voice, to let my own sound come forth. A gut-wrenching groan began at the base of my pelvis, and amid floods of tears this incredible pain began to move. It moved up a little further each day that I worked with it. Finally it moved through my back and up to my stomach, at which point I started to retch and gag. I heard myself uttering a "primal scream" in full force. I felt the sound energy move up through my throat, a total expulsion of fear, anguish, and tension, followed by exhaustion and relief. I had connected with the rage in my bladder and finally let it go.

While the path of my pain was almost chronological, moving a little higher until it finally was out, at the same time I experienced a whole range of events around it that had no apparent sequence. Sometimes I heard myself crying like a newborn, another time I smelled the ether in the mask that was put over my face for a tonsillectomy. I relived the early loss of a male twin and thus began to distinguish between the inside and outside sources of my prenatal grief. I also felt angry that he had abandoned me in an ocean of sorrow and left me to fend alone in a hostile postpartum environment.

Connections would sometimes flow like a river after sessions, faster than I could scribble them down. They had great significance for me, as I began to understand myself, my relationships, and my career from a whole new perspective.

Most helpful was understanding my own anger and dealing with people who are angry and aggressive (as my father was so often). In such situations I can stay breathing and deal appropriately with the incident, knowing that I can later go down on the floor and let myself regress back to the original source that triggered my anger. The charge can be cleared with bodily abreactions, and sooner or later a connection will come and my self-understanding is enhanced. People's anger, I came to learn, has deep roots and a current conflict is usually just a trigger for a reservoir of buried emotion.

Another important insight was understanding that women during labor and birth frequently regress to their own primal experiences, as indeed I had during my first labor. No one else had been able to help me understand why I stopped my labor for almost eighteen hours after my cervix was fully dilated. But for Graham the answer was clear—I had regressed to a primal state—and he proved to be right. I remembered women in labor whom I had observed but not understood. Now I knew.

I became aware that my visual difficulties were my way of withdrawing from what I didn't want to acknowledge in my family environment. I have worn refractive lenses since the age of thirteen. During my primal journeys, I saw how I had chosen not to see, how I avoided looking into the future (symbolic of short-sightedness) based on the original pain of seeing my parents' disappointment that I was not the hoped-for boy. The baby at this stage shortens the focal point so that the mother's face is blurred, setting the pattern for his short-sightedness. *

The most important insights, however, had to do with even earlier memory, as layers peeled off and I went back to my conception and even before, to sperm and egg experiences.

* Myopia, like scoliosis, typically does not present as a symptom until puberty—a symbolic state of rebirth.

CHAPTER SEVEN

The Light at the End of the Tunnel: Making Connections

We can filter reality to suit our level of courage. At every cross-roads we make the choice again for greater or lesser awareness.
—MARILYN FERGUSON

Making connections is the goal and the reward of these inner journeys. It is the experience of reassociating and reorganizing feelings and state-dependent memories that lead to resolution, not just the reliving. Activating resources that were originally denied and utilizing new choices are the keys to empowerment.

Primal pain is not an abstraction. It is above all a sensation, a "bioelectrical force" as Janov termed it. The sensations of our life in the uterus and during birth remain as physical tendencies that become manifest under later stress. When the sensations are chronic or severe enough they can lead to symptoms, disease, and recurrent nightmares. In this way, patterns are experienced over and over again without ever getting to the cause. As in dreams, there are often only pieces or fragmented sensations. "Primals," said Janov, "are the connection of those disparate sensations to consciousness." Lake put it this way: "the crucial task is to make acceptable in our conscious mind the intolerable and utterly unacceptable passivities of the first early life."

Keeping people waiting, needing to work under pressure, and constantly making requests that cannot be filled are common birth scripts that can be the source of constant arguments. In adult life, a person may plunge into projects only to be held back by others who are fearful. Here the surge ahead and the being held back will reawaken unconsciously the birth sequence, and the result will be inordinate rage and impatience. In contrast, aggressive, driving behavior that got one *out* of the birth canal may cause one to die prematurely from overwork or make personal relationships extremely difficult. Similarly, as Janov put it, the "prototypic response of passivity as a life-saving tactic becomes something that can cripple adult life; it inhibits the urge to strive, to function, to succeed, and to be motivated."

Making connections is like finding lost treasures. Contact and connection improve not only within oneself but between others as we unwrap our unopened packages. We come closer to developing a balance among "instinct, intellect, and intuition." According to Groddeck, instinct lies below the threshold of consciousness, intellect holds first place in the recognition of individuals as human beings, and intuition lies beyond both of them "only occasionally making its presence felt in the sudden illuminations and apprehension of truth which are the gift of our greatest thinkers." Johnsen called insight the "emotional intellect."

THE EXPERIENCE OF CONNECTION

People often ask how to distinguish between past reality, their imagination or what they have been told. With regression experiences, our inner knowing becomes more visceral, and certain—ultimately earning our trust. As Montagu explained, once you create your own reality it becomes more real than the unreal.

A connection is information that *dawns*, rather than being chased after or talked or worked out. It may be a spontaneous flash or a satisfying "that's it!" that may arise after days, weeks, or even months. It is confirmation of what an individual knows to be *unequivocably* right, a certainty which an individual has usually not experienced by any other rational or nonrational means of investigation or growth. As one man expressed it:

> I have been and still am a skeptic of the first order. However, through primal connections I understand a little more of the "why" of being me. An important piece of truth about myself becomes mine and it comes from within myself, not from others. Nothing could be more profound or more pleasing. I *know* rather than postulate.

The body doesn't lie, and this profound inner knowing sustains individuals who avoid seeking confirmation from their parents for fear of upsetting them. Also, many mothers erroneously reassure their offspring that the pregnancy and birth were uneventful, but they may have repressed the experience or have been anesthetized.

Bringing blocked feelings into conscious awareness is usually accompanied by abreactions of adrenal and other stress hormones with which the experience was stored. The connection is thus experienced on all levels—mental, emotional, and physical. The physiological response always comes first, then unconscious movement (in hypnosis, the finger or pendulum signals), and afterward the verbal connections. When the memory has been retrieved by the conscious mind, it can be reconsidered and integrated into a person's self-image. This distancing serves to soften the impact of the original trauma. Primal memories remain in storage but without the same blanket of anxiety. The alienated parts of the past have been reworked and regenerated so that the body can become, as Boadella puts it, "charged with the significance of what it has truly lived." There is often a pronounced sense of optimism, as this client expresses:

> I cannot overstate the immense relief and inner peace of self-acceptance I have experienced in uncovering the layers of my past pain, knowing the basis of my intense current pain

and consequent joy of realizing that I do not have to remain
imprisoned by the past, and that I am gaining the power of
choice and change.

As we have seen, hormones work together with feelings, so
it is not so surprising that making connections leads to bodily
changes, such as breast development in women, voice deep-
ening in both sexes, and increased beard and chest hair in men.
Brain-wave patterns of those individuals who have experienced
primal regression in depth show slower rhythms and greater
synchrony, as do those of meditators.

MAKING SENSE OF SYMPTOMS

Grof points out that we tend to live our lives as we lived our
first nine months. He compiled a framework connecting perinatal causes with subsequent psychological problems, such as
depression, substance abuse, migraines, and peptic ulcers; furthermore, he links these birth matrices with social and political
trends.

Any symptoms may have pre- and perinatal origins, but common ones include sleep disturbances, hypertension, anxiety,
feelings of inadequacy and low self-esteem, headaches, backache, lump in throat, nervous skin rash, stomachaches, feeling
emotionally drained, itching, reproductive difficulties, visual
deficits, tumors, immune system dysfunction, and vulnerability
of certain organs.

Sometimes patients have pain in the navel associated with
placental issues, or a compression headache with "steel bands
around the skull" resulting from a difficult birth. Epileptic fits,
he decided, reenact labor. If a connection has been made and
the release of the birth trauma banishes the pains or problems,
then a correct diagnosis is assumed.

Vomiting, including the nausea of pregnancy, is a symbolic
attempt to rid the system of the "toxic influence of the fetus

by expelling it from the stomach through the mouth," literally throwing it up. Ulcerative colitis results when "the too-painful experience has been swallowed and evacuated continually." It is the chronic and inconclusive expression of inexpressible emotions, according to Lake. Cheek found in every instance of gastrointestinal pathology he explored that the client's mother was either unwilling or unable to breastfeed. Genito-urinary problems that seem to originate in later life often result, after a long latent period in between, from imprints at the time of birth.

Obstetrician Paul Brenner had a patient who suffered from anorexia nervosa (self-denial of food). The patient's mother admitted that she had prayed that she would either abort the pregnancy or have a stillborn because they had not planned on a second child so soon after the first. This client had a pattern of seeking out non-nourishing relationships that were short-lived, thus validating her earliest impressions that the universe is hostile and uncaring. It turned out that the woman's mother had fears about being able to nourish her child since she herself had a similar prenatal imprint during her own gestation. And so the generational patterns go on.

Emotional trauma (and sexual guilt) can be converted into a bladder complaint, the bladder being a substitute for the womb. I have long called urine-control problems "urinary tears." Tumors often take the place of a dead child or an abortion, or represent pregnancy fantasies. Menstrual disturbances are an unconscious attempt to release this primal pain through the corresponding part of the feminine anatomy.

I had a patient who suffered from asthma and had *sixteen* nasal polyps removed. The symbolism here is apt; she turned out to have been the survivor of an attempted abortion by her mother. Each little growth in her nose, "hanging on by a thread" (a phrase she used consistently when referring to her marriage to an alcoholic), represented her traumatized inner self.

A client of John-Richard Turner suffered lengthy spasms of hiccups despite years of therapy. Through regression she discovered that her mother had the same symptom during the third month of pregnancy on learning that her husband had been wounded in the war. After these connections were made, the hiccups ceased.

Headaches commonly are birth related and consist of many types. They can arise from natural birth or instruments. Neck tension may be traced to improper head rotation during birth. Migraines differ from pressure headaches because they often result from oxygen loss at birth, coupled with an associated buildup of excess carbon dioxide. Carbon dioxide is a powerful dilator of blood vessels, and that sudden dilation is the chief ingredient of a migraine. Adult stress evokes that original loss of oxygen with all its painful repercussions. For some there is massive vasodilation during asphyxiation in birth to permit the greatest blood flow to the brain, and this can form a protype for migraines in adult life.

Mott believed that asthma has a relationship to the lungs playing a placental role and the breath assuming umbilical sensations postnatally. The asthmatic makes a decision: "It hurts if I breathe. . . . I can't breathe. I'll show them and hold my breath." There is often a paradoxical feeling of "If I breathe I'll die, if I stop breathing I'll die." Janov wrote that chronic asthma can result from temporarily drowning in amniotic fluid, or having the oxygen supply cut off by a twisted umbilical cord, or being too drugged to take that first breath outside the canal. Cheek considers that if a lot of help was given at birth to resuscitate a newborn, in later life such a person can rapidly gain the attention of those around him by developing similar breathing difficulties. Cause and effect, we see, is never cut and dried; indeed, research today is suggesting genetic origins for asthma.

Nasal congestion, bronchitis, and sore throats may all derive from putting a tube down the windpipe to remove fluid after birth. Late breathers experience the shock of air pressure on an uninflated chest. According to Lake, psychosomatic equivalents of chronic resentment and hostility are high blood pressure, ulcerative colitis, asthma, rheumatoid arthritis ("chronic

smouldering resentment and implacable bitterness"), peptic ulcers, dermatitis and other skin reactions, chronic colds or sinus
infections, chronic nasal congestion, and catarrh. In cases of
severe anxiety, asthma, migraine and mucous colitis are seen.
Lake was well aware that "hardened arteries, flatulence, but-
terflies, vague aches and pains, loss of appetite, and "irritable
bladder" are all more treatable to a doctor than emotional
conditions. The physician can slow down degenerative changes
and make the best of residual function—for example, keep
blood pressure down with hypotensive drugs—but this does not
reach the cause. As Janov wrote, "symptoms are hooked into
systems."

We saw already that dreams and fantasies can be tied up
with symptoms. Fodor found that oral birth fantasies may lead
to tonsils, adenoid, and thyroid swellings. He also wrote that
men may be seized with anxieties during and after intercourse,
that "the unconscious mind equates the penetration of a woman's genitalia with the individual's own passing through his
mother." Also connected to birth and before are two ever-
increasing health problems: substance abuse and allergic
reactions.

ADDICTIONS AND ALLERGIES

Substance abuse and compulsive eating or drinking serve to
put an end to confusing states of inside tension and discomfort.
But the solution is only temporary, hence the addictive process.
Ironically, food allergies often go together with cravings. A
person feels driven to gratify the craving, and the allergic reaction will show in a couple of days. Lake suggests that ad-
dictions and allergic reactions can be seen in the same light as
a personality pattern developed in reaction to a "persecutory
womb experience." Denials—especially if strong, as in addicts—demand a life-long mobilization of the adrenal glands,
ending ultimately in exhaustion. The challenge is to overcome

the fear enough to take the risk to dismantle the chronic, maladaptive defenses by making sense of them.

PATTERNS FROM BIRTH AND BEFORE

Many cause-and-effect speculations have been applied to birth. For example, a patient who couldn't quite make it out of the birth canal always sets up situations in which he never quite finishes anything properly. Another client who was lifted out by Cesarean section may never let anyone else set the time for her arrival or departure. Some people allow deadlines for work or study to creep up until there is hardly any time left, then they mobilize themselves into action. Memories of our labor may enable some of us to work well under pressure and to channel aggression into more subtle acceptable forms. Sometimes we are certain that the future will be good if we only try hard enough—which may lead a person to become a visionary. Prenatal ultrasound studies of twins, and postpartum follow-up, have shown that both individual and couple patterns emerge at very early stages and continue to be seen in later life.

Often in regression, an adult will feel that his father's reaction to the pregnancy was negative and feel compassion rather than blame for his mother.

A client described his gestation: "I grew in her fear. When my mother is angry, that is what I am. I cannot separate them from myself." Another's reality was: "I had nothing. I had no connections. It was cut off. And there was just a total sinking into darkness. That started the feeling of being alone, and it just grew from there. At the core of me was a terrible blackness that nothing could change. The feelings seem eternal, endless." Strong desires for an abortion may be communicated to the unborn child, who later may carry fears of destruction or abandonment, and be a loner. One woman jumped into an icecold pool and kept swimming in the hope of aborting the fetus, who turned into an adult who chose to swim in cold pools in winter.

Medical conditions can be linked to birth, such as easy bruis-
ing, morbid fear of being touched, oversensitivity to sight or
smell of blood and anesthetics, colds, fever, or anxieties about
falling, drowning, and suffocation. Cesarean-born adults are
more likely to have rescue fantasies and rely on others to help
throughout their lives. Support can be a major issue for Cesareans; they want help but mistrust possible interference and
that can lead to opposition. Individuals delivered by instruments may seek shortcuts and the easy way out. Those who
experienced forceps and labor-induced infants may have issues
about authority and intrusion. Those who had long, slow births
may become claustrophobic.

Prenatal engrams may cause individuals to go through life
generally feeling unsafe, fearing that someone is out to get them,
or that they have no right to exist. Understandably, there are
problems with trust in relationships. In order to survive, an
unborn or newborn child learns how to be quiet, to play dead,
to be good. Sometimes a "good" baby is so overwhelmed by
trauma that he is in a dazed state for most of his infancy. Having
a history of being passive and undemanding, he might in later
life seek personal relationships that allow him passively to provoke rejection. In work situations he might continually set
himself up for failure. These are all ways to conform to his script
of "Nothing I do will be enough" and "I don't deserve to be
alive."

Ray and Mandel described an actor whose mother had a prior
miscarriage. The actor always felt that he might be the wrong
one, that maybe he wouldn't have existed if the first pregnancy
hadn't miscarried. "In my career as an actor, I find it hard to
take parts away from other actors. I'm guilty when I do get
parts. I never get hired as a replacement, and I live in constant
fear of being replaced myself."

Lake believed that people who experience negative emotions
in the uterus tend to become "night owls" (since when the
mother is asleep, there is less transfer of bad feelings)! Whether
you sleep late or you are an early riser, whether you get ahead
of yourself or fall behind is probably related to birth. Fast births

often lead to living life in the fast lane. Prematurely born people may look upon their bed as their best friend and comforter, becoming insatiable sleepers as if trying to make up for the time lost within the womb.

If some of these connections seem far-fetched, we can look back to an article by Shrevin and Toussing that describes 3 children's conflict over tactile experiences. Written 30 years ago, it is a striking example of how many exciting insights can be lost when the pre- and perinatal model of consciousness is lacking.

Classic metaphors abound, such as "you are the places I have been . . . you remember the tree I brushed against . . . by the river?" "I was born with a rough surface" that came in contact with (her) "mother's rough surface." One child would wriggle around on the floor like a worm saying . . . "I'll just have to kill myself . . . unless I can kill Doctor X," and tried to jump out of a window. Pretence games included: sleeping for extended time, being a dead canary in a cage and play-acting a dirty elephant in order to permit brushing all over.

In these fascinating, but typical, case histories, the authors quite miss the prenatal significance of these experiences as they academically consider "constitutional hypersensitivity" from tactile understimulation and develop models of muscle spasm and myelinization. Rocking and other rhythmic patterns are interpreted as a "compensation for the loss of tactile stimulation which would result from a defensive raising of thresholds."

Temple Grandin describes in her book *Emergence: Labeled Autistic*, how any kind of human touch, even a handshake was intolerable: "it went through my head like a freight train." To enhance her recovery (and she went on to get a Ph.D.), she developed a series of "squeeze machines" modeled on cattle chutes that allowed her to rest inside a box (*uterus*) and feel it compress her body while she controlled levers on a pneumatic device. Reading this much prenatal symbolism in a review led me to order the book, and to disagree with her speculation "that an autistic child's immature and abnormally developed nervous system creates a functionally-deprived environment." I would turn that cause-effect relationship around: she sounds like a classic victim of severe prenatal trauma. Her mother (who is extremely supportive of Temple), was only nineteen when she was born. Temple discusses her *inexplicable* terror of the speech therapist's "sharp pointer" that caused her to "*shrink back in fear.*" As a child she cut up inflatable toys, and would make arm holes so she could wear them on her body. Also, she liked to wrap plastic (*membranes*) around her and was fascinated by museum mummies. Her increasingly severe panic attacks peaked between two and four in the afternoon and made her feel as if she were "clinging to a greased rope (*umbilical cord*) suspended over an abyss." She controlled these panic attacks with her ever more elaborate squeeze machines. However, when the attacks subsided she suffered from eczema ("breathtaking antagonism," according to Hay) and colitis (Hay: "insecurity, difficulty in letting go of that which is over"). During college she became fixated on the Ames Distorted Room (*uterus*) in a psychology book, finally, like with the cattle chute, she constructed a model of it. The turning point in her life was when she "became a cattle chute operator" (she "learned about emotions" in the cattle chute) and "glided through a sliding glass door." In a chapter titled the "Glass Door Barrier," she describes how it took "three weeks of *wrestling*" with a *sliding* glass door fixation to enter a supermarket.

But it wasn't only my fixation on the sliding glass door that distressed me. Using my cattle chute *haunted* me. Outwardly I acknowledged its benefits but inwardly I denied its *rough and harsh origin* . . . the whole concept involved being held. . . . Until I could come to terms with benefit/*rejection* paradox, I couldn't even look at a cattle chute advertisement without *flinching* from the thoughts and emotions which surfaced. It was only after I took a picture of me in a real cattle chute and had it made into a poster and mounted (*made real*) that I faced my fears. Sometimes in the squeeze machine I feel like a wild animal *afraid of being touched*. Maybe it's the fear of opening a door (*being born*) and seeing what's on the other side . . . paradoxically learning to care at the *slaugh-*

terhouse. Designing a "stairway to Heaven" (*birth canal*) for the animals . . . became aware of how precious life was. I thought about *death* and I felt close to God. Using doors as symbols was a fixation from high school into college . . . stepping through a doorway was my means of acting out a decision. (*birth*, *life*) [italics mine].

Today, her panic attacks are kept under control with medication, and she is a successful designer of livestock equipment with her own company.

GETTING BACK IN TOUCH

The skin is the largest organ in the body and also the largest area for sensory experience. Mott considered that "fetal skin feeling" is the basis of the ego. An adult may have a morbid fear of touch from loss of amniotic fluid prior to birth (the maternal environment was rough and irritating) or mishandling at the time of delivery. Sometimes a strong dislike of touch arises from being washed and rubbed, and then weighed on a cold scale. Loss of touch makes one fearful of contact and yet ironically creates a deep need to be touched.

My mother was very young and not ready to care for a baby. . . . I know she did not want to hold me because I always feel that people don't want to touch me, that there is something wrong with me. I know that all my life I have been looking for the bonding that I never had, so I expect too much from relationships.

Epilepsy, tics, stuttering, and sex are ways people discharge tension. What many people want out of sex is actually touch rather than sex. They desire the warmth, protection, love, closeness, and reassurance that touch brings and the price they are willing to pay is sex.

Problems with the umbilical cord can cause a person to feel cut off at the neck from feelings below. There may be an imprint of having to struggle by pushing and pulling back. Brenner mentioned the case of a woman born with the cord around her neck, who had experienced a feeling of shock whenever she was emotionally distressed. She later developed malignant lymph nodes in her neck.

Twins may suffer from separation trauma. The one left behind feels angry and the one who left first may feel guilty. If the second twin was undiagnosed and thus unexpected at birth, he may go through life feeling, "Nobody notices me. I am an afterthought. I shouldn't be here." He often feels that the first born is treated as older brother and he is second-best. Maybe there is an imprint from the mother that the first baby is the one she wanted and thought she was having; the second, then, is the other, the "extra." Twins, after birth, are invariably separated from each other as well as from their mother.

Postpartum separation from the mother can lead people to feel their entire life that they need to be alone and separate in order to survive. They may become resigned to the motto: "I can't get what I want. . . ."

Breastfeeding helps the baby recover from the ordeal of birth. But sudden weaning, warns Fodor, may "reactivate the dim organismic imprint of the violence with which the child's body was wrenched out of its mother." The time of weaning often proves to be a critical period during which the "psychic and nervous future" of the child is determined. This may manifest itself in breast fetishes, compulsive smoking without pleasure, and even kleptomania. Love and food are synonymous and interchangeable in the unconscious mind, and there will always be a "yearning for something unattained, something missing" in the pysche of the bottle-fed child.

RESISTANCE AND RELATIONSHIPS

The first assumptions we make concerning ourselves and our relationships often form the context for future choices in relationships. The conclusions we carry from birth and before form an "unconscious legacy." These "personal laws" make us live the opposite. For example, if you think you are stupid, you will act smart and try very hard. But if you are always living in fear of being discovered doing something stupid, there is little satisfaction or safety in your intelligence.

Turner called our attention to the "law of opposition" and warned that what we resist will persist. He called this the "law of confirmation"; that is, "What I believe about myself, I'll keep proving to myself." "As long as I resist, I'll keep going through it." For example, to the extent that we feel we need someone in order to survive, we will subconsciously push that person away in order to feel self-sufficient.

People who experienced obstetric intervention (painful support) during birth may equate help with pain, and go through life saying "I'd rather do it alone." Birth was the first big change in our lives, and it affects how we make changes. Being born was a liberation, but it was also a separation into the unknown, and at this time our sense of adventure is either kindled or crushed.

Prenatal imprints may cause a person always to be moving on, having to get out of situations, apartments, jobs, and relationships and sometimes at regular intervals. Many relationships and many jobs end after nine months.

Ray and Mandel described one of their staff members who was put in an incubator for almost three weeks. She explained the effect on her relationships:

I feel a sense of urgency over where the relationship is headed—almost as if having to reach some kind of completion as soon as it's begun. I very much feel that I have to wait for me to be ready to love me, and I have to stay separate from them when intense, loving feelings, especially mine, come up in the relationships. I notice that the time I always think is appropriate is some where between two and three weeks; then I can be with them again.

GOODBYE TO GUILT

Adults often feel guilty for causing their mothers pain during birth; they may have developed a theme of always ending up hurting the ones they love. Men who believe that they caused their mothers distress, according to Cheek, are overly apprehensive when their wives approach the time of labor. Lake explained that the unborn baby may feel compassion for his mother's distress and even begin a lifelong role as "fetal therapist." Bearing stress and coping in such a situation allows the unborn to gain some degree of confidence; in later life, I believe, such individuals may choose the helping professions or do a lot of volunteer work.

Peerbolte was one of the first to observe that female patients often experience their own feelings from prenatal states during pregnancy and birth of their children and project these emotions on to their children. He describes a woman whose mother died during birth from a retained placenta. She showed the same symptom in her three births, with danger of hemorrhage.

Forgiveness of self and others comes when we can let go of guilt and remorse, which follows when the pieces of the puzzle fall together and we understand the bigger picture.

STARTING EARLY

Emerson first saw the potential benefits of helping infants regress in 1974, when he was asked to consult on a case concerning an infant girl whose severe bronchitis had not responded to medical treatments. Emerson's therapy included massage that simulated birth pressures. Interestingly, at the moment when the infant's head "emerged" she began to wheeze, although similar pressure on other areas of her body had not evoked any response. This experience was repeated several times, and again on subsequent days. Each time when she pushed herself out, the bronchial episodes occurred but diminished in intensity, until the last session, when there was just a deep sigh. At a twelve-year follow-up, she had no recurrence of symptoms.

In contrast with adults, the success of treatment with infants depends on the extent to which the primal feelings are *contained* with touch and contact, and to the degree that deep contact is made between the parents (or therapist) and the infants.

According to Emerson, from the age of about two and a half to three and a half there is a perspective of distance developed, a "spectator self," although severe trauma can disassociate the witness. The corpus callosum that connects the two hemispheres of the brain is not fully developed until age seven.

Emerson once helped a toddler who went into a state of terror when approached by his father and showed extreme anxiety toward strange men. Sand-tray work revealed that he identified closely with the figure of a battered unborn baby. After Emerson described the boy's reactions of being beaten and tortured, the mother started to sob, "How did he know? I never told anyone, not even my husband." It turned out that during the early part of the pregnancy she had an extramarital affair with a man who threatened to "beat the life" out of her if she didn't leave her husband and marry him. On several occasions he dealt violent blows to her body, including her uterus. However, the toddler—in just four sessions of regression therapy with both parents present—was able to release his emotions from the prenatal abuse. His symptoms of anxiety around strangers and his ambivalence toward his father disappeared; after several years he showed no signs or side effects of the abuse.

The problems of 45 of 75 infants referred to Emerson for behavioral disorders (such as sleeping or eating problems, ir-

ritability), emotional disorders (crying, fear, lethargy, with-
drawal), and medical conditions (including colic, asthma,
eczema) were successfully resolved by primal therapy, and 66
when medical treatment was included. Emerson pointed out
that if parents can recognize the emergence of primal pain, they
can see their infant's behavior as therapeutic and thus be more
able to support the infant and affirm the behavior, instead of
complaining that the baby is fussy or difficult.

PIECING TOGETHER THE PUZZLE

A first step is to explore the present stress that reactivated
the primal emotions and triggered the symptoms. "But," mused
Lake, "doctors of sick bodies are not usually qualified to be the
doctors of a sick society and of broken personal relationships."
As both a missionary and a psychiatrist, Lake noted that both
religion and medicine repress rather than confront anxiety. The
limited time and lack of training in both fields narrows our
concept of mental health to just the absence of troublesome
symptoms.

The representation of autonomic functional upsets as "illness" becomes a "behavioral technique in order to reach
inaccessible love objects." They are simply part of the human
condition and have nothing to do with doctors or real diseases
even though they can be described in medical or quasi-
medical terms. Only their fixation, leading to chronicity and
their separation from the emotions which are still, in depth
causing them, leads to this threatening state of affairs. The
danger is that if they are not heeded when used as sign
language, and attended to as communications of otherwise
inexpressible ontological needs for better relationships, they
may well go on to permanent pathology needing medical
attention.

Louise Hay, author of several books and tapes on healing, has written a handy little reference book, *Heal Your Body*. She lists hundreds of symptoms, from baldness to constipation, and cancer to rheumatoid arthritis, suggesting their symbolic significance and offering an affirmation (positive statement to counteract the negative thought behind the condition). It is the exploration of therapeutic possibilities that is important here, rather than an attempt to classify diseases or to squeeze experience into a narrow framework.

After exploring the current issue, the next step is to pursue the earlier and earlier experience of, for example, "not accepting the self" (acne), "longing to be held" (aches), "feeling of futility" (alcoholism), or "not wanting to be a woman" (amenorrhea, or lack of menstrual periods).

The following story illustrates the process in a person who was not merely curious about her past but had been treated for "mental health" problems:

My name is Mira. The first half of my life was spent in total pain; the second half belongs to me. I was thirty-two when I discovered primal therapy. I searched all my adult life for an answer to why I was "chronically depressed." I made my outer self into whatever people wanted me to be: always kind, considerate, friendly and agreeable, never angry, annoyed, unpleasant or bitchy. Yet in all my life I'd never formed close bonds with anyone, male or female, never developed any special directions. I was so deathly afraid of physical contact or emotional ties. I tried one therapy after another, this doctor then that one, drugs, a psychiatric hospital, even God. Finally there was nothing left to try. I could no longer ignore the little girl, me, who "appeared" in my room night after night, wringing her hands, shoulders hunched, eyes begging for help.

It's been six years now since I started having birth primals. Sometimes I had ten or twelve before any connections were made, the first being that a "part" of me is missing. I dance beautifully in my head, I can hear the beat, but I cannot move my body to music. I attribute this to literally being forced from the womb, my sense of rhythm destroyed, when my mother took a very large dose of castor oil three hours before I was born.

Another connection made was why I always delayed starting anything new or important. I missed out on a great deal because of this, and even though I knew it, I could not stop myself from insisting on my terms. When pressured as to why, the only reason I could give was that I was "not ready." I had to be in control of the speed of events, had to have plenty of time to prepare myself for change.

My first minutes in this world are very vivid in memory, being left flat on my back on a cold surface, the incredible weight of my body from head to hips, unable to move beyond my arms and legs thrashing wildly in nothingness. The world I'd known, dim and supportive, was suddenly gone, changed into noise and light, bright redness and yellow, and cold, cold white. I was left there to scream alone in horror and terror because, the nurse said, my mother had to be "cleaned up" first. My first experience of being touched by another human being was when the vernix was literally scraped from my body, the skin that one moment felt so cold, was now burning, tingling, and twitching. (Until I felt this in regression I could not bear to have my arms touched and the feel of cold air was enough to turn my limbs to jelly.) I could never understand why it made my navel ache and why my vision was cluttered by a brilliant red haze.) They pried open my fingers and wiped away the fatty deposits there, the last familiarity I had, the warm feel of that vernix in the palms of my hands. All my life, when faced with a situation that was likely to be unpleasant or beyond my control, I made sure I had something, usually a hanky or a tissue, clutched in the palm of my hand.

The big traumas I found easier to reach, such as being orally raped at the age of two. When I first relived this one, it lasted three days and three nights, and connections came thick and fast. That's why my teeth rotted one by one till at fifteen there wasn't a sound tooth left. That's why I'd had one cold sore after another. That's why I suffered from sore throats and bronchitis. I never let myself be loved or let my needs be known after that—to need meant death.

When I started to write my experiences of regression I thought, yes, that will be easy. But now I find that I can't remember much of my first primals, dramatic though they were at the time. This, to me, is proof that primaling really works. I've felt so many old and early pains and now they are gone. I no longer act them out. I can't say that I am now completely free of pain. I'm not and I still primal occasionally. The difference is that now I know what is happening to me when old pain comes up and I can deal with it. I'm no longer afraid of me or afraid to be me.

Sexual abuse, the lamentable experience of a majority of young girls, is a very common recollection in age regression and often results in multiple personality disorder.

LETTING GO AND MOVING ON

Making connections is thus central to the process of reliving early experiences. The ultimate connection to be made in regression is with one's "real" self—the self that was whole before it was split, before the heart core was abandoned. Inside experiences help people rediscover their own reality as they travel to usually painful, and sometimes blissful, past events.

An invaluable part of the connection process is the emotional relief and satisfaction that results from making sense of symptoms and feelings. Freud noted, to his great surprise at first, that hysterical symptoms disappeared after they had been brought to memory and described by the patient. However, instant cure is more of a myth than a reality.

Insights do not always immediately relieve symptoms; sometimes numerous reexperiencing of the early trauma may be necessary. Not everyone is able to simply let go of issues and undergo a radical change. * However, as Sufi master Meher Baba stated, "the individual never achieves true freedom until he is no longer pushed or pulled by any inner compulsion."

Healing is more than just making a connection. "Making whole" leads to greater coherence among thinking, feeling, and action; a felt purpose in life often emerges. Thus, healing acknowledges the soul, which was experienced along with the heart as separation. Feeling more authentic, secure, and calm, integrated individuals find less interest in competition and in driving themselves to meet former goals. Instead they become attuned to the here and now. As author and TV personality Leo Buscaglia put it, "Yesterday is a cancelled check, tomorrow is a promissory note, today is cash—spend it all you can." Once the step has been taken to live in the present, it becomes easier to transcend the self and experience spiritual dimensions of existence.

* I know why I wear refractive lenses, but I have been lazy and inconsistent with eye exercises.

Conception Revisited

Nature prepared us to be radically more creative, intelligent, and powerful than we currently are. Why aren't we?
—JOSEPH CHILTON PEARCE

A single cell like an amoeba, we learned in high school biology, can exhibit learned behavior. It is clearly "conscious." A gamete cell (egg or sperm) is carrying far more DNA—indeed, the whole genetic code of the parent plus all the knowledge to start new life. From conception through birth an individual develops through the most complex system of creative intelligence that has evolved in the universe. However, as Lake warned, "when 10^2 million embryonic cells have grown to become 10^{62} in an adult, each seems to have passed on its tale of woe to its now extensive progeny."

Since most people do not even accept the idea that babies remember birth, it is stretching the limits of their belief to discuss memories of conception and before. However, in mystical scriptures of the East, intuitives have pondered the metaphysical aspects of conception for centuries. The ancient religious notion of the sperm as *numen* (a spiritual force) and conception as *numinous* (filled with presence of divinity) gives credence to the experiences that are described in this chapter.

In the old Christian tradition, the pneuma or spirit is called the *pneuma spermaticon*. In our own culture, there have been at least a couple of physicians who have written on this topic. Georg Groddeck wrote in 1923:

I go so far as to believe that there is an individual consciousness even in the embryo, yes, even in the fertilized ovule, and in the unfertilized one too, as well as in the spermatozoon. And from that I argue that every single separate cell has this consciousness of individuality, every tissue, every organic system. In other words, every unit can deceive itself into thinking, if it likes, that it is an individuality, a person, an "I."

The recording of one's own conception suggests the presence of a soul. Peerbolte asked which "mind" records the three facts of fertilization—egg, sperm, and their mutual attraction—which consists of perhaps an "extrapersonal or cosmic libido." The fact that ovulation, conception, and preconceptional states come up in dreams shows a psychic relationship between a woman and her ovum, postulated Peerbolte. There is clearly a relationship between the fertilized egg and the corpus luteum (the yellow body in the ovary that secretes a hormone after fertilization to secure the pregnancy).

FERTILIZATION

Attributes to gamete cells, such as "resistant egg," "tired sperm," may sound unreal, and unscientific, but the spontaneity with which such images pour forth gives them a striking imprimateur of authenticity.

Conception depends on hormonal conditions that sometimes give rise to an "outpost fight of maternal and paternal hormones." As Peerbolte puts it: Impotence, premature ejaculation, and "aggressive forces" from the father have a hormonal effect on the egg. The ovum has to bear the pressure of mother's psyche, including hormonal disturbances around ovulation and menstruation, all of which can affect the balance between ovum and sperm, as well as function in the oviduct. Delayed implantation may also result in postconception bleeding, which causes insecurity in the egg.

The relationship between ovum and mother is more materialized contact than the relationship between egg and sperm. The mother's original knowledge about her egg is transferred to the egg itself during or after conception, which becomes the root of telepathic prenatal contact between mother and child. Gender desires of the mother are usually clear to the individual at the time of his conception.

The hyaluronic acid within the head of the sperm facilitates penetration of the egg. The fear of losing one's memory is connected with a too rapid dissolution of this cell in hormonal fluid. There can be a "precipitate penetration" of sperm, with the excess male hormone surrounding the egg and causing "vehement fears and even depersonalization."

Peerbolte compared the process of conception with an electric current. Electric tensions and directions of the current are dependent on the conducting qualities of the hormonal layer. The two poles of egg and sperm result from the first reduction division. The hormonal conditioning of the egg determines whether this first reduction division will be experienced as an expulsion or primary castration with the cell being driven out by sperm, or if the tension between these poles will be harmonious. The principle of order and regularity (such as symbols of clock and time) represent the ovarial aspect, in contrast with "an illogic principle, the libidinous aspect of the spermatozoon which cannot be understood in an intellectual and ordered manner."

SPIRITUAL ASPECTS OF CONCEPTION

Ovum and sperm are in some respects carriers of an energy that stands apart from both matter and the two gametes. This energy is indivisible but in a sense it has been split into male and female by its crystallization. Noetic qualities, life principles, as well as prematernal feelings and the attraction between the male and female cells may all be present at conception, according to Peerbolte's speculations. He also felt that female sexuality can often be activated only in a kind of "spiritual sphere." The attractive force is the "root of all sexuality, one of the basic elements of the human psyche." As Reich also observed, the energetic qualities are very great whereas the actual matter involved is very small (two cells).

THE EXPERIENCE OF CONCEPTION

Rarely is there a perfectly balanced and harmonious union of sperm and egg components. Therefore it is not uncommon that one gamete feels victimized by the other, was engulfed or invaded by the sperm, or recalls a struggle of reluctance or outright resistance from the egg. There may be an experience of parental ambivalence concerning conception, the man having perhaps second thoughts as he ejaculates and so the sperm shoot forth to their goal but carry seeds of doubt. One woman's description of her egg as "paranoid and apprehensive" and her sperm as "critical" reflects her perception of parental emotions. Likewise, another man complained, "I have difficulty with sexual feelings from having taken on my mother's sexual repulsion during my conception." Peerbolte found that depersonalization associated with a denial of the sexual sphere in conception can cause frigidity in the offspring's later life.

Sexual determination can be a traumatic event because the primary sexual reorganization, male *and* female, results in a corresponding psychic imbalance: the resulting zygote is either male *or* female.

Fertilization involves the union of the largest cell in the human body, the egg, with one of the smallest, the sperm. While some sperm are triumphant, some straggle along reluctantly in awe of the great round orb. I recall one man in a workshop describing how he saw a huge golden ball, which chose him by rolling over on top of him. He also connected to the fact that this is how he perceives his relationships with women. Christopher felt himself as a struggling sperm, arriving close to death and being overwhelmed by an "omnipotent, emasculating egg." This connection enabled him to successfully revert from his homosexual orientation. One woman described her conception as taking in a sperm, while having the feeling that there was a better one for her somewhere out there; this was also the story of her marriages.

A woman in Australia described her sperm journey and its continuing effect on her life:

> I am a sperm in my father's testes. I am being jostled, frenetic energy in and around me. I need to go to burst out of here. If I don't I will implode and die. I was conceived on my parents' honeymoon. My father's feeling is intense excitement and urgency. My mother is terrified and resistant. At the moment of union there is both force and outrage. Their feelings are the blueprint for my life: my mother's rage at my rape of her, in passing through her body in birth—father raped her from the outside, I tore her from within. Every year in June, the time of my conception, I become frantic. I want to go, just go, anywhere, fast. The house, city, and state are all too small. None of my friends, relatives, people on the street give me any room to move. My anger is profound and my head wants to explode. I have done many journeys at the beginning of winter fearing I would die from the cold. I once moved myself 2,000 miles north to be nourished by that beautiful large, golden, pink sphere—my sun egg.

Meg's experience of her conception was quite different from her mother's experience: "Mother perceived it as rape but my father was out to enjoy himself . . . a happy eager sperm wanting to join, but finding a terrified egg hard to 'get through'."

An astonishing reality of "sperm truth" caused one of Graham's clients to question his "father's" paternity, which led to the eventual tracing of his biological father on another continent! One woman primaled a completely different sperm experience from the rape conception her mother had always described. She subsequently found her father, reversed her attitude toward men, and was able, at the age of twenty-six, to have her first relationship with a man.

The "death" or loss of identity, of egg and sperm is a necessary part of fertilization, as the gamete cells merge in a new creation. As one woman expressed it, "I've had a sensation of needing to shake off a tail—a sperm feeling. I feel the need to disintegrate in order to be made whole." Peerbolte suggested that acceptance of conventional death, theologically, may be interpreted as conversion, or a conscious acceptance of conception and thus birth and rebirth.

The egg is commonly perceived as all-knowing and wise. "The *power* I had as *one* cell to affect my environment I shall never have again," mused R. D. Laing. However, Australian physician Christopher Millar noted, the egg lacks the facts to externalize this wisdom, "like a programmed computer with no data to operate on." A woman after one of my guided visualizations wrote:

> My vision of me was the egg, round, free, glowing. When you came to the sperm my vision became one of surprise and shock. Yet, I felt the sperm were invasive beings. The surprise was that I needed this to happen in order to create life. My attitude was, "What are you doing here?" Nobody told me I needed this! I wanted to take this journey "freely." Well, that was my first disappointment, the prerequisite of that sperm for life.

People who result from an unplanned conception may feel that they have no right to exist. They go through life apologizing: "I'm sorry to disturb you." "I'm sorry to interrupt." "Do you really want to invite me?" At a cellular level, they feel guilty for taking the option of life.

Not infrequently, an individual in regression experiences an explosive buildup of pressure in his head, as if it were going to burst. This is indeed what happens during fertilization as the genetic material is released into the egg. Although headaches seem obviously related to birth, I suspect that many may be connected with conception, especially when they come on in situations of union or conflict. I once treated a minister's wife for a gynecological problem, alongside which we did some exploration of her feelings (without any mention on my part of the possibility of primal memories). After her first session on the floor (during which she reproduced a lot of typical sperm movements and mentioned her bursting head), she sat up and exclaimed, "You won't believe this, but I felt just like a giant sperm!" Her "splitting headaches" were related to the experience of division after fertilization.

Sperm primals are typically characterized by a lot of foot and leg movements, and butting of the hips, rather like the actual flagellum which lashes back and forth to propel the sperm forward. Sideways movements of the hands may also indicate sperm experiences. When I watch a person's foot twitching during conversations, I often wonder if they are experiencing an old sperm memory . . . and becoming anxious if they are going to get in, in this case, into the conversation.

Persons reliving their conception may feel absolute terror of penetration. Unwanted conceptions, such as during rape, are often experienced as gagging, retching, even spitting up the unwelcome invader. Amazingly, such individuals often end up in situations of abuse again and again in their lives. Residual primal pain causes people to unconsciously manipulate their environment in order to avoid, or create, conditions that facilitate reenactment. As Graham has observed after facilitating thousands of people, for twenty years in eight different countries, human beings are motivated toward health. "We create situations in adult life," he explains, "to gain resilience over the trauma of cellular consciousness, not to masochistically suffer repeatedly."

Millar wrote about the lasting effect of the experience that results from the interaction between the sperm and the egg: how the egg is affected by the presence and behavior of the sperm, and the sperm by the egg. Each will have their registration at the gamete level, and the fusion of the two affected gametes results in the "curious situation in which the physical entity constituted by the zygote is now carrying the memories of the interactions of the two entities that produced it. Thus we are simultaneously that which was done to us and that which we did to another. As Millar explains:

> It's almost as if I chose myself: how I wanted to be, what I wanted to be, what I should look like, what abilities I wanted for life in order to achieve what I set out to do.

Laing divided his life into three stages: A) conception to implantation, B) implantation to birth, and C) his postnatal life, demonstrating where he felt the major influences lay—two-thirds uterine.

I observed and later interviewed the following client of Graham as he relived his conception experiences:

> I believe in cellular memory—anything that intense has to be real. I recall being the ovum leaving the follicle and entering the red fleshy tube. It was like being carried on an escalator. I was terribly uncomfortable, nauseous, and I didn't want to be there. It was all foreign. I don't like caves, and escalators "get me"—elevators are okay. I have to close my eyes, I have a sense of things moving past me. [He gestures with arms circling and sweeping over his head representing the hairlike cilia in the tube.] I feel the threat of the endless tube and lose my sense of my physical body, feel I am going into another world where I don't belong [he claws his navel]; something poisoned me here. I have a sense of the placenta being reversed, and my mother wanting some thing from me. I have all this confusion about in and out again. [His mother wanted a man in her life.] I always had problems with my own space, felt invaded, people cutting in, wanting part of my body.

Adam described his pre- and postgamete consciousness:

> My sperm feelings are like being enclosed in a piece of music, waving, jackknife movement, feet together like a tail, movement all the way up to my head. My powerful, tense back

is the central experience. I always want to move right through the middle of the room. I must take the center path with no obstruction. Letting go feels fantastic, if I'm rigid there's no chance. My egg was calm, centered, circular, with a wall holding everything out. I experience blissful feelings at the end of such a primal. I accept myself; I am aware of beauty in movements, like dancing on the floor, feelings of expansion, lacking barriers yet centered, at one with self, omnipotent—a light, total feeling.

For people like Cathy, staying with the feeling itself can be a real act of courage:

I don't seem to be able to ever sort out what's going on with me all the time. It's just like I fell over and can't get myself back up again. Down into the roots of it, I am beginning to understand that just maybe there can be an end to it, to my hell. I can't make myself respond; the fuse has gone, there's no connection, I can't plug in . . . nothing but anguish, despair. My feeling is "the egg has nothing to give the sperm; it's not worth the struggle. I feel a terrible loneliness; it's not a good place, this is not what I am supposed to be. My own feelings never line up [classic sperm metaphor] with what I meet. My conception was just the beginning of an endless process of being told I am wrong, not just a local fact but a whole fucking existential reality. I've seen the same look on children's faces. I'm terribly afraid of letting anyone see me weak and hurting. I need to stay in touch with the divine part of myself, which I could never see before I had primal therapy. It was a blind spot [wise and knowing egg].

Rosemary, who was orally raped at age two, connected this to her "fixation" on oral sex after she left home at age eighteen: "In oral sex, I'm in control, on top. I'm going against the tide, like when I was a sperm, washed backward." She recalled her earlier primal experiences:

My egg prior to conception was full, radiant, light, blissful, and separate. I felt the sperm looking up to egg wondering, "Will there be a place where everything is fertile and I'll be myself?" I felt connected, without any barriers. I experienced a creative environment to "be me": relaxation, bliss, and peace.

Mine was a violent conception during the honeymoon. I felt very deep, completely, totally "in" the feelings. The egg was seductive but didn't want penetration. When it happened, there was a feeling of outrage. Implantation meant no place for me, not getting enough nourishment, feelings of choking on my mother's fear and revulsion. My mother was similarly conceived; her mother's husband raped her on their wedding night.

Kathy experienced a fuzz around the egg, a grayness and fog that she had to get through. She explains:

I felt nothing in particular; I was somehow not activated. I needed a sperm to feel a different entity. But I couldn't see him; I tried to reach him on the other side. [Her father was drunk during the conception, thus a possibly toxic sperm.]

Eric expressed the same experience of "inside and outside" as R. D. Laing described:

Feeling is inside, the intellect is on the outside. I always wanted to know what makes life tick. I didn't get the feel of me because I was always observing how I live life instead of living it. Now it is almost the reverse. I want to live and don't want to know. I start with the thought and I play it out in body, to get to the truth of the body.

I became aware of generations of pain—not being able to get close to people. I experienced a sensation of needing to shake off a tail and a need to disintegrate in order to be made whole. Getting in touch with the lovely bouncing and wafting of the egg, deciding whether to implant—"I can decide how I can live"—gave me an enormous sense of power. I felt part of another force and an enormous cycle, which is very reassuring. I am now tuned into people's simple unmet needs and hurts and see how they are driven to other things.

The few fortunate individuals who were created in love and harmony re-experience a blissful merging and one-ness. As Sarah described it:

I experienced a great stillness and no physical movement before a still quiet sperm. Then I had a feeling of being the egg, dancing. After the sperm had finished turning the egg, I now began the journey on my own, a beautiful feeling of completeness.

Other people retain more impressions of splitting than union, and often go through life using the phrase, "Part of me feels. . . ." They tend to have "splitting headaches" or feel "divided" or "torn in two" on issues.

Graham created the first documentary of "conception revisited" in adulthood when his own experience was filmed in 1979. At that time, he did not understand the symbolism of his movements, most of which he cannot reproduce voluntarily but only in an altered state of consciousness. The activity of the cytoplasm going out to draw in the sperm is clearly shown by Graham, as he circles his arms in a symmetrical, embracing action. This phenomenon was observed several years later in the laboratory (in a microscope slide the cross section looks like two arms).

Ten years after Graham's first personal experience of cell division, the exceptional NOVA documentary, *The Miracle of Life*, showed how the fertilized egg pauses before the two first cell divisions. These biological photographs both paralleled and confirmed Graham's reenactment of his own conception.

Brenner holds that men and women are simply "eggs and sperms with delusions of grandeur." He sees the male psyche and its expression as myth in our culture as one of fear of loss of identity, inevitably resulting from the death and destruction of the sperm during fertilization. Male knowing, wrote Peer-bolte, is an "aiming at" in contrast with female knowing, which is "feeling, being at one with." Women are born with all their eggs and a deep sense of the continuity and sacredness of life. Brenner explains that men build arms and fight wars because they believe that after death there will be resurrection, as in their prenatal experience. In contrast, women offer contain-ment and fear abandonment. Their ethic is survival, needing the energy of the male, just as the egg is started on its journey down the tube by sperm energy.

REPRODUCTIVE TECHNOLOGY

By definition, assisted conceptions require more than nature can achieve by itself. In the early 1940s, Alan Guttmacher, a famous U.S. gynecologist, made a pioneering (albeit facetious) observation about artificial insemination with husband's semen. He remarked that "if the sperm need a boost of several centi-meters to help them reach the egg, won't they be too bashful when they meet it?" Graham speaks of "reluctant gametes" mixed up in a test tube where they can't escape from forces that otherwise would not have brought them together. The comparison has been made with medical care; if we left every-thing up to nature, then many diseases would not be treated. Therefore, we must have a "war on infertility" (defined as the inability to conceive after a year of trying) like the "war on AIDS," for example. However, the analogy has quite different ramifications. Reproduction involves the creation of a new being who will carry the emotional imprint of that creation for the rest of his or her life. It is too early to know yet if adults who develop from frozen sperm have issues with cold, or how light affects gamete cells in the laboratory when under normal circumstances their labyrinthine journey is entirely in the dark. And as for embryo transfers, the thought of being flushed out to move house at such a critical phase of development is terrifying.

Although some infertility support groups do offer workshops on the mind-body connection, I suspect that they are not oriented toward gamete consciousness. Texts and congresses on infertility never seem to link the condition to the brain. Infertility is always perceived as a problem with the reproductive organs. Medical professionals simply give the label *idiopathic*, which means "without known cause," to diseases that they don't understand. In Chapter 12, I describe how one of my clients resolved her infertility (habitual miscarriage is classified as infertility) through the connections she made after regression to her embryonic experiences. Behavioral approaches are as successful as drug therapy in many cases and without side effects. Often regression is the *only* way to resolution.

Sometimes women are told that they have "hostile cervical mucus," and doctors attempt to create a more favorable environment for the sperm with various drugs. It has happened that when cervical mucus from such women is tested in the laboratory, donor sperm swim through but the partner's sperm are blocked! Amazingly, the cells in the mucus can differentiate the origin of the sperm, probably via resonance.

Unbelievable as it sounds, there are women who have finally conceived with donor insemination (DI), or *in vitro* (IVF), or gamete intra-fallopian tube transfer (GIFT), only to demand an abortion. These cases understandably infuriate the medical staff who assisted at these conceptions. Consciously, such women may have believed that they wanted a baby, and familial and social pressures can be overwhelming, but when the baby became an internalized, organic reality, they realized this was a major mistake.

Counseling for assisted conceptions, especially third-party or collaborative reproduction, is essential. It is usually inadequate if it exists at all; more money and attention are paid to technical wizardry. However, because our conscious mind is responsible for only about 10 percent of our functioning, couples with infertility, especially if no organic cause can be found, often need more than counseling. By delving deeply into their primal scripts, these individuals can find out first if, at their innermost depths, they really *want* a baby and then explore the biographical, and perhaps intergenerational, issues that are preventing success.

Prenatal Dynamics, Generational Patterns, and Life Scripts

We shall not cease from exploration
And at the end of all our exploring
Will be to arrive where we started
And to know the place for the first time.

—T. S. ELIOT

My primal issues began long before birth. It was the reliving of my conception, in individual sessions with Graham, that provided the most fruitful insights and helped me toward greater self-awareness and change.

My father, so the family tale goes, was unplanned and unwanted, and conceived when his father was intoxicated. Grandfather was already an irremedial drunk and little Dick came into the family long after the five other children, to be raised by his eldest female sibling. His mother at forty-four (the age I was approaching when I had my son) had her hands full with six children. Lack of bonding with his own mother, and insecurity in his own masculinity, was at the core of my father's contempt for women and his striving to endow his two daughters with as many male skills and attributes as possible. Since understanding that my father was a victim of profound and unresolved primal pain, I have been able to feel sympathy for his behavior after decades of resentment.

My singular memory of my stiff and aged paternal grandmother is that her remarkably large ears had pierced lobes. I had never seen anyone with holes in their ears and they made a big impact on me. Of equal significance was the one and only

fond vignette painted by my father of their relationship when
he was a small boy. Grandmother would let him climb onto
her lap and reach up to place a pin through the hole in her
ear. The significance of this came home to me when I understood cellular consciousness: he enjoyed feelings of easy and
successful penetration!

Such a metaphor for conception is made even clearer to me,
as I carry the ambivalence of my father (creating a third girl)
and meeting strong resistance in my mother's frightened egg. I
have always felt that life should be a struggle, since I struggled
with the conception and later with the decision to breathe (to
take in life) in the uterus after the death of my twin and my
sister.

But there was an earlier, gamete feeling from the time of
fertilization. My sperm-self expects resistance, which I can set
up from my egg-self. This has meant much wasted time in
relationships and activities in which I lost my vision in the
process of struggling. If I had been better integrated and more
in touch with my core self, I would have felt free to make
changes a lot earlier.

On an intergenerational level I have also linked this conception dynamic with Julia's loss of an index finger. At age
two and a half she placed her finger in the open hole of a
compost leaf grinder that Geoff was using, and it was completely severed. Children do like to investigate holes, but in
my family the significance was profound. I believe it was a
memory of my father piercing the hole in his mother's ears that
she carried unconsciously. I also connect this pattern with her
conception by artificial insemination, and a symbolic desire
(unconscious, of course) by my sterile husband to cut off the
power of the donor (his penis). (It is interesting that among
his extended family, there are at least two other cases of loss
of a finger. In contrast, there were no cases in my family
history.)

I made all these connections in a matter of minutes after
one session; they just popped into my mind like pieces in a
puzzle coming together.

THE BLADDER AS A
SEAT OF EMOTION

Just before my labor began I had been reading Wilhelm Reich's *The Function of the Orgasm*. It could not be mere coincidence: my unconscious mind must have absorbed his description of an "armored bladder"—the stretching of the surface membrane by the constant production of internal sexual energy (contractions)—and the "rigidification" of the body preventing the bursting.

According to Hay, bladder problems represent "anxiety, holding on to old ideas, fear of letting go, and being pissed off." Those adjectives describe both my mother's demeanor and my labor. (My mother would never show her anger, nor would she have ever used a phrase like "pissed off"; she was as tight-jawed and puritanical as my father was scatological and explosive.) As I paced around the small primal room at Graham's clinic, I lived again the pelvic paralysis of my labor. All the anger and unwept tears concerning my conception were stuffed to bursting into my bladder.

After accessing my gamete memories, I characterized my labor with Julia according to insights from my early consciousness. The first stage of labor was an "ovum experience," a circle opening, the roundness of the egg—my cervix, her head. The circles grew bigger with contractions and I enjoyed feeling stretched to my limits, but yet still retaining those boundaries.

When I-as-egg started traveling down the tube to meet the life force of the sperm, I became incapacitated with terror. This was the linear, descending energy of the second stage, and as soon as I felt the power of those contractions, I wanted desperately to STOP. The male force of the sperm, I-as-sperm, came up again and terrified the egg part of me, triggered also by unexpected resistance from my husband to calling the doctor. I froze completely, determined not to let anything in or out. Baby and urine—all held back, with blocked breath and tense sphincters, as the egg tried to keep the sperm at bay. It was a complete feeling of "No! I don't want this. I don't even want to be here in this universe." The moment was enormous; labor and birth were distant points on a far horizon.

I think if someone had said to me after the contractions stopped, "What are you feeling? What do you think your body is expressing? Let's talk to your baby. Let out some sound" (as I had during dilation), perhaps I could have pulled out of this regressed state. I was so split that my intellect was functioning exceptionally well and no one recognized that the other 90 percent of my consciousness was dangerously shut down. As a result I fell into the pit of unscientific obstetrical nomenclature that typically labels labors that become dysfunctional for non-organic reasons as "failure to progress" and "uterine inertia."

Urinary functions had a high profile in our family. My mother always told me that I was "such a sweet little baby" until I went to the hospital and "contracted cystitis" (inflammation of the bladder). Although I was born at home, because that was not the plan, an ambulance nevertheless took us both to the hospital for the customary ten-day "lying in." Perhaps my mother had a urinary tract infection at the time or else there was contamination in the nursery. My mother had a long history of frequent urinary tract infections.

My father always teased me about my "pint-sized bladder," which incidentally never would last through a movie, and any time when I was anxious I would void frequently. (The word void also means "to make empty," symbolically to empty out feelings.)

Since my intensive primal exploration I no longer experience any nervous need to empty my bladder, and during my second labor I didn't even have time to think about voiding. The birth was quick, easy, and painless! The bladder drama of my first labor had thus been completely resolved by making these connections.

GAMETE IMBALANCE

I see that throughout my life I have fluctuated between the terrified egg and the ambivalent sperm. The egg provided the structure for the sperm struggle. "When you make your bed," my mother always preached, "you lie in it." I always perceived my mother to be a fearful person, although she did stand up to my father's brutal insults with stoic pride. I am also able to stiffen up and resist attackers in arguments like my mother or my egg. In fact, when I am outraged, my perseverance knows no limits. Often, however, my mother opted for denial and would pretend not to have heard, say, if my father farted loudly and deliberately in front of her bridge group, or insulted her in front of the gardener. Her response was resistance—not letting it in.

Sperm energy has been my driving force on many levels. I first experienced that incredible life thrust, together with considerable existential reluctance, in a workshop with Stanislav Grof. My partner, who was a psychiatrist and no means a novice in this situation, tried to help by "birthing" me. One of the facilitators made an equally inappropriate stab with his finger into my navel. However, all the while I was undoubtedly experiencing myself as a sperm—driven but full of doubt—toward the huge egg cell. My approach in this particular session involved bending my body backward, under the egg in a way that made just a partial border of the egg visible. I was able to draw this image quickly and clearly in a mandala after the workshop. It was a feeling of slipping over a horizon, perhaps also falling onto the planet. These same feelings come up very powerfully when I see a photo of the earth taken from the moon. I don't like to live inland; I prefer to live on a coast, with a horizon on the ocean or a border on a lake—as I drew in my scene on the first day of my intensive with Graham.

A surprising revelation to me was that my partner, during that regression to sperm, insisted that I went backward, not forward, while I had an indisputable sense of leading with my head! It is still hard for me to believe that each time (and I did this five times) I led with my feet. My rational mind then questioned if this was really a sperm memory, since my knowledge and training told me there was no such thing as a "breech" sperm. For successful fertilization the head of the sperm has to enter, and it does so because its "hat" of enzymes dissolves the protective layer around the egg. I did not know then that scientists have since observed sperm trying to enter eggs tail first and even sideways. Also, many sperm get waylaid in the tube's crevices on their journey to the egg.

THE LINK BETWEEN A "CONCEPTION SCRIPT" AND FERTILITY

On a subsequent visit to Melbourne I had a session with Graham to explore my sensation of thickening around my hips. I had also been trying to get pregnant for several months. As a child I was irritated by the sound of my mother slapping her thickened flanks when she was in the shower—supposedly to improve their muscle tone—and this memory came back very strongly.

Graham softly suggested that I let myself feel how it was to be the egg. This was something I had not yet experienced. I immediately went into a very deep state of absolute terror and recoil. "Sheer terror" were my actual words, and later that day I coincidentally went shopping for pantyhose and I was struck by the connection that *sheer* meant "filmy, vulnerable, letting in light." Feeling so *sheer* made me want to thicken my zona pellucida (the inner cellular layer that surrounds the ovum), and symbolically I was doing that again with my adult body, wanting to be pregnant at one level but fearing conception at my core. I also connected with my egg memory of that same thickening in a futile attempt to prevent sperm penetration of the zona pellucida around the egg.

Women resist conception in many ways: tension in muscles

that close off openings—inner thighs, buttocks, pelvic floor sphincters; thickening of the flesh around the hips and buttocks, stiffening of joints; or sometimes just sensations of the reaction without actual bodily changes. At the other end of the continuum are women who will not consciously plan a pregnancy, but throw away birth control and "let it happen." Sometimes, part of a woman wants to know if she is fertile and ovulates with orgasm. (I believe I did this with my first pregnancy that I aborted; the timing was at the end of my cycle.) Whatever the conception dynamics, they reverberate through the life of the individual and often can be better understood in a generational context.

Several years after I became conscious of my zona pellucida experiences I was sitting in a living room in Houston, surrounded by strangers and a medium who channeled an entity named Father Andre. When my turn came, Father Andre made the profound statement that I was "afraid of being penetrated by the male energy at a cellular level!" This was one of the most amazing insights I have ever experienced. I am still astonished! It was so true for me and yet so different from the kind of remarks he had made to the others.

Later I came to understand why I had chosen (unconsciously, of course) my first husband, who ten years after our marriage was found to have *no sperm at all in his semen*. My unconscious gamete memories left me too afraid of sperm and made sure I wouldn't confront a single one! Ironically, my husband's sterility obliged me to experience donor insemination, which required much more handling and proximity of sperm than during a sexual encounter! (I have written in detail about this experience in my book *Having Your Baby by Donor Insemination*.) After I had done several unsuccessful inseminations, an infection in my cervix was diagnosed. I saw through the microscope that one lone sperm was completely choked off by a mass of white blood cells, a symbolic zona pellucida. Since I never had any clinical symptoms of an infection, I believe this was a functional response from my body as a result of my inherited ambivalence concerning conception. Wanting a child was a strong desire, but there were barriers formed as a result of my conception dynamic. (I did take antibiotics and conceived after a couple more inseminations, but the real issues were not addressed.)

Four years later I tried to conceive a second child with donor insemination, but gave up after several attempts. The loss of my daughter's finger, and its many deep associations with my primal pain, plunged me into a state of grief that lasted more than two years. My husband, while understanding my desire to have another baby, was at a loss to find a direction in his own life. This lack of purpose that I perceived caused me to feel more and more resentment toward him. I didn't mind providing financial support for a few years—in my opinion, everyone has the right to take time out and to change a career. But I was reaching the limit of my ability to keep on giving. Bringing home the bread as well as the sperm made me feel as if I were "wearing the pants." The primal imprint of "I should have been a male" clashed with my growing female desire for motherhood. As those feelings grew stronger, the struggle inside me grew more intense until I knew the only solution was to break free, to *get away* from the situation, as I did at birth.

Although I was glad to leave my mother's grief struck uterus and enter the world, I knew I would confront my parents' disappointment at my gender. Likewise, leaving my marriage and going into the emptiness of the unknown was frightening, but ultimately healing and empowering. The survival skills that I had learned prenatally helped me find strength during the couple of years I spent alone. I took risks and found greater riches, including a new relationship and a naturally conceived son, which I describe in my forthcoming book, *Channel for a New Life*.

BIRTH SCRIPTS AND CAREER CHOICES

We have seen that symptoms and life scripts that result from prenatal experiences can be understood and resolved through regression and making connections. Reality, we must always remember, is an individual construct, and what is true for one person may not be the case for another even in similar situations. Also, as therapist Anne Wilson Schaef, Ph.D., pointed out, "recovery is a process, not an event." And this event is often ongoing.

I believe all of us seek our professions for some karmic reason. Those of us in the medical and paramedical world, however, have more responsibility to discover our primal motives because the well-being of our clients is in our hands. The man who fixes the telephone wires may have primal feelings about umbilical cords, but he does not affect parents and offspring as intimately as a midwife or obstetrician.

My most dramatic insight occurred at a large international childbirth convention where I had led a group of about eighty in prenatal exercise. For closure, I guided a brief relaxation session with everyone lying on the floor. I gave just a few suggestions such as: "Allow yourself to go back in time . . . to when you were floating in your mother's uterus. Become aware of the predominant emotion you felt from your mother. . . . Did you feel that you initiated your own labor and birth, or did events happen to you?"

As I directed their awareness back to the present time, one movable wall of the room was being opened up for the thousand registrants who were streaming in for the luncheon banquet. People clustered around me and it took a few minutes before I realized there were still some people lying on the floor. One woman had totally regressed to her "second-stage arrest," quite incredulous that she had experienced a phenomenon of which she had always been highly skeptical.

Several weeks afterward I received some hostile evaluations of that brief experience. One in particular stood out: "I know I had a horrendous birth and I don't want to know anything about it." This is precisely the challenge of this field for most obstetricians, midwives, labor and delivery nurses, and childbirth educators. The susceptibility of the conference attendees to regression was heightened by their having spent several days and evenings immersed in birth issues. I knew this from having helped midwives and childbirth educators regress after other conferences. If this is how a birth conference stirs their primal feelings, what about the effect of assisting at a long and difficult labor?

As a result of these experiences, I made two very significant conclusions that profoundly influenced (and continue to confirm) the direction of my life's work. First, it showed me that maternity-care providers indeed do have more unresolved pre- and perinatal anxiety (and more burnout) than the general population. (There are exceptions, of course, but they tend to be just that, exceptions.) How ironic that the experts usually have the most complications when they birth! Second, I realized that no matter how many studies, how much research, how many "hard facts" are compiled in favor of natural birth, interventive obstetrics will continue until providers can be freed of their unconscious, compulsive need to interfere (albeit with the best of intentions).

Many of our birth scripts have been influenced for the worse by the insensitivity of those who attended us when we entered the world. Frederick LeBoyer had already observed that violent births resulted from a situation where there were "no monsters, no sadists. Just people like you and me. *People whose minds are elsewhere*" (italics mine). As a result, in Chamberlain's words, newborns have been "traumatized, trivialized, and depersonalized."

Moreover, with advances in prenatal screening today, those outside influences reach sooner and deeper into the sacred space of the womb. I suggest that pregnant couples ask how their maternity-care provider was born. Find out if your doctor or midwife was premature, induced, delivered by forceps, or Cesarean and so on. What victim experience prenatally led them to work in a helping profession? What is their rescue (Cesarean, instruments) rate? You will be able to evaluate them by either their response or their resistance! And if you are giving birth in the hospital where you obviously have not personally selected your labor attendants, you will need to have compassion for them when their unconscious birth memories are aroused and their support becomes replaced by anxiety.

IMPLANTATION

Most of us know people who will never ask directions, but will circle around, get lost, and be late, instead. This behavior often relates to a primal feeling of ambivalence in the fertilized egg about reaching its destination.

Many people recall a state of bliss prior to the attachment to the uterus—feelings of cosmic consciousness and interconnectedness. Even in unwanted pregnancies, conception and journey down the tubes can be pleasurable experiences. Implantation is the first time we connect physically with our mother, and this can be a rude awakening if she does not want to be pregnant.

> Mine was a blissful conception of soft egg and a gentle sperm. My pain began at two months when my mother became aware of pregnancy—feelings of constriction. My mother emotionally denied pregnancy and physically constricted it. My bodily experience was a bone marrow, skeletal level of pain. It took enormous life force for me to grow each cell. When I am overloaded now in daily life, the same pain returns.

Rolando Marchesan reported about a woman who at fifteen days after conception "felt a light tension which did not allow [her] to be completely at ease." Her mother told her later that at the time she was worried about losing her job.

Fortunate individuals experienced a warm reception, like sinking into a luxurious red plush sofa, while others found a resistant uterine wall. If fibroids were present, they perhaps had to search around for a space and had to burrow in. Implantation actually does involve fingerlike projections of fetal tissue that take root in the wall of the uterus.

Powerful imprints result with regard to acceptance or rejection. In fact, a mother's first reaction to her pregnancy is the most significant marker for the child's future self-esteem. If her feelings are negative, as Cheek so aptly puts it, the fetus feels as if he has been invited to dinner and then asked to leave when he arives. Growing up confused and troubled, he will tend to reject his mother or distrust her demonstrations of love and acceptance. Some people in later life suffer "implantation terror," sensing that other people don't like or want them, and worrying about their reception when entering a room full of people. Implantation, remarked Laing, is a "template for all reception, entering pushing oneself in or being pulled in, battling one's way in or a reciprocal embrace of love."

Some of Michael Gabriel's clients described this situation:

> From her standpoint, my mother was thinking "I'm pregnant, but I don't want to be pregnant. I don't want to face my mother over this." But I took it personally, like she was saying to me, "I don't want you" . . . like her rejection of me was blaring over a loudspeaker.
>
> My mother has found out she is pregnant. When she realizes this I can no longer remain outside. A connection opens, and I am immediately pulled into her body. It's as though her awareness sucks me into her body. I lose my separateness, I am part of my mother now, without a sense of myself. It's as if you could see right through me.
>
> I felt so dark, empty and unwanted during the prenatal period. I think that's what produced that deep feeling of emptiness I have now.
>
> That seems to be the key decision of my life, the decision that my mother didn't want me, that's been the guiding feeling of my life.

Donald had been seeing a chiropractor twice a week for almost two decades prior to moving to my area. He had painful muscle tension in the left side of his body, specifically his left shoulder. I told him at the outset that I would not continue physical therapy treatments without improvement. For the first couple of sessions I worked traditionally with massage, ultrasound, and exercise and when I was finished he felt worse! (I understood this as his need to hang on to his symptoms.) He was curious when I asked about his birth; I had thought to myself that perhaps his shoulder may have gotten stuck during birth, knowing that the more chronic the condition, the earlier the cause. Donald knew he was conceived just before his father left for the war, because his parting words to his mother were, "Get rid of it before I get back."

When Donald arrived for his third visit, he was emotionally charged about a recent conversation with his mother, and most resentful of her reticence to share information. I encouraged him to lie down on the floor right away and explore those feelings as deeply as possible. Soon he was on his front and groping all over the room. Clearly he was not in a birth primal; he was looking for a place to put down his roots. Part of him eventually gave up—the left side—and pulled in. The limbs on the right side stayed outstretched. After attaching as best he could, he rolled onto his side and lay there sucking his thumb. He later made the connection that the pain and stress of implantation split him in half. When under stress, his whole left side, especially his upper extremity, tightened in the same way. After this session he also noticed that his constipation (holding on to old ideas, being stuck in the past) was much improved as were his shoulder spasms.

By repeating the past we do unto others as was done to us. One woman described the intergenerational effect of her implantation:

My egg experiences my mother's bleeding as I try to attach, to implant. As a result, while I know I am going to make it as a spiritual entity, physically I don't feel I will: the life force of knowing but a physical reality of dying. I later conceived a child during my menstrual cycle, too.

Life is often a conflict between isolation and engulfment, a struggle between the desire for freedom and the desire for security—struggle that has its origins at this time:

I had an incredible sense of floating in the tube, choosing to stick on, to live. Implanting meant giving up the free rolling, but I knew that not to do so meant death. So the next step was to trust my mother to look after me for that length of time. Realizing that I had a choice was very frightening. I've always had a problem with commitment in all areas. In some ways I am free and mobile, but a part of me dies if I don't stick on. This is such a real feeling, it's really obvious. After birth I cried so loudly in the nursery I was finally put with my mother so I could stick on.

RELATIONSHIP WITH THE PLACENTA

Babies have been observed, with ultrasound, stroking the placenta and burying into it like a pillow.

Laing wondered if it were possible that "patterns of giving and receiving, going and coming, imports and exports" are registered before birth. He noted that now he needs an alcoholic drink at exactly the same time as his birth, 5:15 P.M:

> Many people feel they have never been born. Others feel they have never been implanted. Others are just implanted, unreconciled, pining, mourning, crying for the moon, the ghost of themselves as blastula before burial in the womb.

The navel represents the solar plexus, the "brain of the sympathetic system that responds with dangerous facility to thought," wrote theosophist Annie Besant. Chronic abdominal tension can develop from trying to keep something out that was coming through the cord. There can be confusion between the female-mother and the placenta as bloodsucker, destroyer, and place of death which can carry over into pathology in later life. We resent people who are "sponges," or who are "tied to the apron strings," especially when we didn't get enough! The placenta makes a singing sound and I wonder if those people who hum to themselves are experiencing their happy placental memories.

WRONG GENDER

It is very common for individuals, usually females, to feel themselves to be the unpreferred gender, even back at the time of conception. There is a deep primal conviction of being a disappointment and even flawed. Sometimes it is obvious—the fifth son or the fourth girl, or names that fit either sex, like Lester or Robin. I can recall women who were called Christopher and Toby. One client explained to me:

> I felt consciously that Mother wanted a boy and Father didn't even want another child. I couldn't just float in the uterus; instead I felt choked. Mother was always critical and misunderstood. I never felt protected and I felt sad and cheated when my father died. After primal therapy, my breasts grew because of hormonal changes when I became more accepting of myself as a female. My whole body is more feminine, and I have bought more feminine clothes.

Both men and women who were the unpreferred gender may have difficulty accepting their true nature, and this later influences their preference regarding the gender of their unborn child. I have held workshops for expectant and new parents that delve into issues about the gender of their offspring, and I was surprised at how many enrolled. People have gender preferences for a whole range of reasons—cultural, familial, logistical, religious, and emotional—and they must be explored, not denied. Typically, such expectant parents choose *not* to confirm the gender of the unborn.

Cheek found that if a mother didn't know (under hypnosis) the sex of her unborn baby, "it was fear in about 100 percent of cases." Fear will cause abortion in animals in early pregnancy; in human labor fear shuts down the cervix, despite contractions. Sixty percent of miscarriages start at night, according to Cheek, after dreams containing transient anger toward the husband or a member of his family.

Many gynecological problems such as cystitis and vaginal discharge can be traced to a sense of feeling unwanted as a female at the time of birth. Cheek warns that:

> it does not matter how much love and acceptance are shown later. The child will imprint on such remarks as "we wanted a boy this time" or "we did not select a name for a girl." Such children distrust subsequent shows of appreciation and always have trouble accepting compliments graciously.

I could never accept compliments from any source. "Let them in" is a conception dynamic. I would always be embarrassed and disbelieving of any appreciation, and my response would consist of excuses, denial, and self-depreciating apologies. I became a workaholic and an overachiever to prove my worth to my parents.

Women who undergo amniocentesis and do not choose to learn the sex often are putting off "bad news." Barbara Katz Rothman, in her book, *The Tentative Pregnancy*, reported that women who underwent an amnio felt fetal movement later than those who didn't. She also found that while women who learned that they had a boy *at birth* were usually elated, those who learned *in pregnancy* that they were carrying a boy tended to be disappointed. Although Rothman did not pursue the deeper reasons why women were not happy to be knowingly pregnant with a male, as Graham points out, "it is a challenge for a lot of women to walk around for nine months with a penis inside." In other words, it is related to the mother's experience of her own conception: how her egg accepted the sperm, the other, the male energy.

My parents so wanted a boy that their wishes were telepathically conveyed to the family doctor. When I obtained my mother's medical record, I found that the event of my birth merited a mere three words: "BBA (born before arrival) *Male* Infant." Just before she died, I asked my mother if she and my father had chosen a boy's name for me. Despite the verbal difficulties from her strokes she replied without hesitation, "Yes, Christopher"! Yet I was not named for several months and referred to as "the baby" in my mother's diary.

I wanted a daughter as my first child. I was not ready to share another prenatal experience with a male. This was a significant step in healing my "wrongness" at being a female, especially since I did conceive a girl. (I guard against expectations on my part that she carry projections of my unconscious wishes, fantasies and ambitions.)

REPLACEMENT BABIES

I have always felt it must be uncomfortable to be named Junior, or the III, a nomenclature that affects only the males in our patriarchal society. (I recently met someone who was the "5th"—a very tall, imposing man with a booming voice, all of which I am sure he needed for his identity to survive as number five.) Far worse, however, is the burden of existing as a replacement for a child who died, and especially if named after the dead person as well. The uterine experience in such cases is usually one of a grieving womb. Survivors of a multiple pregnancy often feel responsible and guilty, especially if the death has not been openly acknowledged in the family.

Eileen, who was conceived to replace an older dead sibling, lamented that she never felt she was herself. It was always "I and the other one" (dead sibling). She felt she was "never good enough, could always have done more, been more, given more." She had a long relationship with an older man who died, and suffered chronic guilt that she couldn't have done more to keep him (a symbol of her dead sister) alive.

In a reversed situation, I know a family where the death involved an infant twin who was named after the father. Two years later he was still on medication for depression.

BIRTH DEFECTS

The unborn baby asserts himself in different ways. He causes hormonal and other physiological changes to make the pregnancy possible, especially since he is a foreign body, otherwise his mother's immune system would reject him.

Some birth defects appear to be a conscious choice on the part of the baby, and this information may reassure many women who feel there must have been some sin of omission or commission on their part when something is wrong. They rack their brains over what might have caused the defect, disease, or dysfunction. One of Graham's clients owned his intent in creating his deformity.

I was born with one club foot, which I deliberately twisted in utero, to gain love and attention as I was an unwanted pregnancy. I was born by Cesarean so my experience is commonly one of a lot of initiative but no followthrough. I often have good ideas that don't come to fruition. Still, there is a streak running through me, a knowing that something is unequivocably right. This is the missing piece of the jigsaw puzzle that I am here to explore. It almost rocks my being.

Why would there be a conscious choice to develop abnormally? Here we get into spiritual beliefs. Many people, especially those who have relived such choices, suggest that the baby chooses his burdens, like his parents, for the soul development required in this lifetime. Sometimes retribution is in order. Psychic Edgar Cayce, for example, said that gay people today are people who were intolerant of homosexuals in a past life. Others who were rich in a past life get a turn at being poor and vice versa. Physician Gladys McGarey describes dreams and insights that parents had about their "special children" in her book *Born to Live*. One mother said:

I blamed myself at first, thinking it was some thing I did or didn't do during my pregnancy, but woke up to realize Tara's message to us was, "Hey, this has been my choice, you know. You have no reason to feel guilty."

Another mother had a dream in which she was told "This was not done to you. It was done *for* you."

LIFE PATTERNS

Many individuals discover that major experiences occur in specific time cycles in their lives, and these are related in most cases to prenatal events.

Beverly is a woman who had set up a pattern of "threes" after her twin died in utero at three months. She moved house in three-year cycles, and her births were all three weeks overdue. She was sexually molested and attacked with a knife at age three. Beverly didn't tell her mother, who was then pregnant with her brother, for fear it would harm the baby. When Beverly later became pregnant, she had a Cesarean, perceiving surgical delivery as another surrender to a man with a knife, for fear that something would happen to her baby (repeating her mother's pattern). Her hands were tied down for the Cesarean just like during the childhood rape. She concludes, "I didn't want to want to look at the loss of my twin, or an abortion I had later (after which I developed gall stones). Instead, I suffered a Cesarean as a tradeoff." (Gall stones symbolize anger; "what gall—I could throw stones at you.")

In *Voices from the Womb*, Michael Gabriel includes prior levels of consciousness, soul journeys to earth, incarnations, personal evolution through various realms of existence such as intentional miscarriages and stillbirth.

Alexander Lowen wrote that "knowledge becomes understanding when it is coupled with feeling." Whatever we unravel in regression—personal laws, scripts, generation patterns—the knowledge and the inner knowing bring relief and resolution. As we change ourselves we also liberate those around us and help our children to live freely in the house of tomorrow.

Womb View: My Uterine Influences

We have pushed so much of our life away, held it captive so deep within us that when we begin to let go we notice how much our expectations, conceptions and preconceptions have limited our experience.

—STEPHEN LEVINE

During my mother's second pregnancy she contracted rubella. At the time, she was unaware of any symptoms and therefore not prepared at all for a special-needs child. Anne was severely affected, but my parents did not realize that she was blind until several weeks after birth. (In those days they thought babies didn't see anything for the first few weeks.)

After two subsequent miscarriages I was conceived. Because of my mother's history, and spotting in early pregnancy with me, she went on bed rest, and received progesterone injections from her general practitioner. I remember that my mother would say how much she wanted me, and I know when she saw I was normal, she did, despite my being the third girl instead of the much-desired boy. However, truly wanted pregnancies, I now understand, do not need medical interventions to sustain them. I lived awash in her fear and ambivalence and I didn't understand its source. The contradictory messages of her reality versus mine created a "double bind." An ongoing consequence of this during my years at home was my interpretation of my mother's counsel as "the opposite is true." Having developed a strong survival sense, I was also very resistant to criticism or advice: I raged against life. Knowing from the beginning of my existence that I was the wrong gender, I was determined to feel "right" on just about everything else. I admit that I continue to enjoy standing up against wrongs in the environment, especially when they affect the unborn, newborns, and women.

My mother explained that they had to send Anne away because I was coming. Anne went to the Institute for the Blind in Melbourne, where she later died, without being reunited with her family again. This was practically all the information that my parents ever shared about her. Occasionally, on the anniversary of her death or birth, my mother would become tearful and mumble something about Anne, which would send my father into a rage. He would tell her to "Shut up," and then either she or he would leave the room with a loud bang of the door.

My nephew, Richard, was born twenty years later exactly on Anne's birthdate. Tactfully, my sister delivered two daughters, like her mother, before her two sons. This avoided competition with Mother as well as potential jealousy on the part of Father. Rick, like me, was the third child but the first son. He represented the symbolic fruit of our father's thwarted desire, and significantly was named after him. His arrival on Anne's birth anniversary, I feel, was an opportunity for healing family wounds of death and wrong gender that unfortunately was never taken up.

My father always indicated that he considered Anne's death a great relief for everyone. A handicapped life and the financial strain was over. But "relief" without grief—adequate mourning—was an issue that came between my parents during their whole life together.

TWIN LOSS

I figured that the overwhelming sadness that I had felt inside my mother was a result of her losing Anne. However, in one primal I had the experience of watching an embryo being sucked down and away, swirling into a vortex. In later experiences I had clearer images of that lost twin, seeing one side of his face and one eye before the embryo floated away (an age of about six weeks according to the identical appearance that I later saw in Lennart Nilsson's photographs of the unborn). This was also the origin of my terror over blood.

My reaction to the early loss of my twin, however, was overwhelmed by the experience of total immersion in my mother's anxiety (over whether she would miscarry me, whether I would be normal) and her ambivalence (if I were not normal, then miscarriage might be a good idea), and her repressed grief over Anne. All these emotions were compounded by the global anxiety in 1944 about World War II. My mother's deep fear at my conception is quite understandable. She was approaching her fortieth birthday when I was born and had already borne a child with congenital defects. She knew she would greatly disappoint my father when she produced yet another girl, and would blame herself (unconsciously, of course) for the lost male.

I didn't understand the all-pervasive nature of her sadness until I procured Anne's death certificate and calculated that *she had died when my mother was six months pregnant with me.* This I had never known; I had always thought it was sometime when I was a child. By then a mother myself, I felt an anguish that moved me to a deeper level of understanding. Compassion for my mother welled up inside of me. I began to comprehend the intense and extensive effect of Anne's death on me. By the time I was making these connections under Graham's facilitation, my father had died and my mother had suffered a couple of strokes that left her with a severe speech impediment. In the last few months of her life she tried to express her pain. Her eyes would fill up with tears and the most she could ever sputter was, "I had a blind baby who died," waving her hands in desperation, asking for help and acknowledgment but also gesturing that she wanted to push the reality away. I consider it symbolic that my mother's stroke caused problems in both the language center of her brain (dysphasia) and also the muscles involved in speech (dysarthria). It was as if her body made sure that even at the end, blocked communication at every level would never allow her feelings to escape. For years she *wouldn't* discuss it, and then when she wanted to, she *couldn't.*

Since then, I have learned much from women who have

grieved the death of a family member while growing a new life, and from expectant mothers who have lost a twin. These are extremely painful, tearing-in-two situations. My mother suffered a similar paradoxical situation of having to both mourn and bond, to allow feelings of loss as well as of joy. It suddenly struck me why I had written a book *Having Twins*, focusing on multiple *pregnancy*, although at the time I had no idea. Ten years later, in my revised edition, I included a chapter called "Emotional Consequences of Twin Loss" for the surviving twin, mother, other siblings, extended family, and the rest of society. Significantly, I was unable to write that chapter, which involved many interviews with grieving parents, while pregnant with my second child. I determined not to repeat my own prenatal experience and create a generational pattern by subjecting my unborn son to an environment of vicarious sadness.

Unresolved grief continued to haunt our family. When I first became pregnant, my mother did not tell anyone, she was so apprehensive about a bad outcome. My mother's response when my daughter lost her finger was, "She must never know that it happened—don't *ever* tell her." Such were her powers of denial. My sister's comment after the accident was, "Well, she's still got nine other fingers," a redefinition of the reality that does not support the loss. Interestingly, Anne was born with six fingers on each hand.

Our family dynamic is thus one of totally denying not just feelings but even events. The lesson here for me has been to completely honor and respect another individual's reality and to learn compassion, a quality I felt to be markedly absent in my upbringing. Since my first experience of regression with Eva Reich, I have on many occasions got in touch with my despair in the uterus—an environment of unremitting sadness. I met Geoff in India after and after a brief sojourn together we went our separate directions for several months. During that phase, I sent him two "funny" cards: "You and me against the world!" and "How can I love you if I don't know where you are?"— both twin loss metaphors, I now see. Long before I read Frank Lake, I *knew* what "negative umbilical affect" was. This led me to choose a husband who was like my mother, agreeable and accommodating but emotionally unavailable on a deeper level. Thus I ended a clandestine, nurturing, and exciting relationship that had begun in my early twenties with a man thirty years my senior. The dynamics of our relationship did not allow the reenactment of the lost twin scenario. This unique individual was not just the obvious father figure but a substitute placenta! He gave all of himself, in every way. But unused to such constant flowing love, I couldn't let it in. Invariably, I would be embarrassed and disbelieving of his loving gestures and compliments (my old prenatal law, "the opposite is true" or "I can't be any good, I'm not a male"). At a cellular level I did let him in once, and became pregnant. In shock, I didn't hesitate to have an abortion and postponed my grief over that event for a decade. The pain surfaced when I realized I had aborted a passionate conception to marry a man who turned out to be sterile.

Decades later I realized how I had sought this ghost bond of my twin in relationships. My boyfriend when I was at University was building a boat to sail around the world, and of course, away from me! As my mentor astutely pointed out: "You didn't want *him*: you just wanted him to want *you*."!

Unlikely Links

There are always surprises the deeper one digs down into the primal memory bank. A couple of years after my intensive in Australia, I was organizing a workshop for Graham on Cape Cod. Logistical problems centered on the loss of electrical cords; I had brought the coffee maker and the projector down from my office in Boston, both without their cords. I cursed the manufacturers' designs for having detachable cords, but later that day I lay on the floor and got into issues with my umbilical cord. I used to suck my thumb to make up for the cold, dead cord; my mother put my hands in bags and tied them to the crib.

I further explored my feelings about the umbilical cord in a workshop with Michael Irving (see Resources). Blindfolded, we were given a cordlike length of wet clay. Mine felt so freezing that I could hardly hold it. In fact, I inquired if the clay had been refrigerated! Others in the group did not find their clay cold at all, but I hated working with the dead, cold, heavy, lifeless "turd."

I wrote the following poem:

> Dead chain
> Cold links
> No movement
> But eyeblinks
> Sick torsion
> Rising tension
> Pain and effort, but I'll do it.

When Michael asked us to cut our own cords, I severed mine fast and furiously! I don't like drawn-out farewells to this day.

Laing wrote that "the world is my womb, and my mother's womb was my first world." Novelist Henry Miller went even further:

As far as I can make out, there is never anything but womb.
. . . It is failure to recognize the world as womb which is the cause of our misery, in large part.

As a child I banged my head, which for me was "Knock, knock, is anyone there?" because I grew in an uterine morgue. I continued to experience issues related to my "first house." Despite a recession in Massachusetts during the late 1980s that caused thousands of other people to have a residence for sale for as long as I did (three years), the base feeling for me was nevertheless primal. Down on the floor it was *an old house that won't move just like my mother's uterus: empty, dead, a burden. I*

am powerless, I can't make anything happen. Since I believe we
are creators rather than victims of external circumstances, I
wonder if there was a karmic reason why I again fell into this
situation, beyond the depressed real estate market.

I am now living in a house of my own design. Like so many
women, I moved during pregnancy—implanted—in a new
nest. To build a house, with light, space, and room for movement (exercise room, primal room, decks) was an integrating,
satisfying accomplishment. And water. I am surrounded by lake-
front views and bordered by woods. For years I have indulged
in an outdoor hot tub. At last, I have the perfect uterus. And
my favorite hobby is ballroom dancing—joining with a partner
(my lost twin) and moving to umbilical cord rhythms.

Individuals who enjoy good relationships with their mothers
may be puzzled if they experience negative emotions in the
uterus during altered states of consciousness. Confusing feelings
may lead them to believe they were unwanted, having been
conceived too soon after a miscarriage or death of a sibling, for
example. In contrast, their experience of their mother as always
loving and accepting may well be the case; many unplanned
babies are wanted by the time of birth. But a negative prenatal
imprint can be a barrier to deeper intimacy. Sometimes the
unborn baby feels in some way responsible for his mother's
depression or resentment, which may, in fact, have nothing at
all to do with him but be related to external influences in her
life. Making connections untangles the lines of communication
within families.

Despite my experience of a sad and anxious uterus, and the
double standard that I always felt existed between my mother's
feelings and reality, she was always my preferred parent. She
protected me from the sarcasm, rage, and violence of my father
and she supported my dreams, even the one to "get away." And
I have lived the major part of my life abroad, the early years
spent travelling alone in search of the ideal male (twin) union.

CONTINUING CONNECTIONS

The greatest benefit I have found from regression is that I can do it any time to find out the original source of my fear, anger, or whatever emotion is triggered by a situation in my daily life and thus continue to build my self-knowledge.

For example, when I was going through my divorce, my husband delayed signing the papers to transfer the car into my name. At this time I noticed my gums became sore: they itched and ached for a couple of days. I lay down on some pillows to feel the sensations as totally as possible. Soon I felt the need to scream and bite. I bit into a pillow, with immediate relief. I continued to bite, visualizing my teeth sinking into my husband's back, when all of a sudden the image shifted to my father! The old pain of powerlessness emerged. (I did not want to be powerful, just simply empowered, and there is a difference between these two states.) My perceptions of my father's aggression (and he was very aggressive by anyone's standard) and my husband's passive aggression had the same effect on me: I felt victimized. I had been told that in my childhood (and I remember the spankings) that I bit other children. At that oral stage the teeth are an effective means of aggression for a child. I traced the feeling of powerlessness underneath the need to bite to an even earlier origin—in the uterus—of being unable to turn off my mother's grief and fear. It is also symbolic that a pillow in a pillowcase represents a baby in a uterus, and I vented my rage at the level of my uterine experience.

As I sat through the 1991 Polish movie *The Double Life of Veronique*, I became progressively convinced that director Kryzstof Kieslowski must be a surviving twin. His prodigious use of reflections, mirrors, views through windows and double images is striking, and apparently not limited to this particular film. Further pre- and perinatal symbols abound, such as a couple making love in a passageway in a rainstorm (amniotic fluid bursting in the birth canal), and the unique style of a singer, echoing a range of notes reminiscent of placental sounds.

In the story, an unknown man tries to attract Veronique anonymously with middle of the night phone calls and by shining beams of light with a mirror into her apartment. This pursuer had noticed her in the audience of his puppet show in which a ballerina broke her leg, was buried in a casket and reborn as a butterfly. He sends her several "clues": *one* shoelace (the missing part of a pair, and a symbolic umbilical cord, which she immediately puts in a washbasin of water), an empty cigar box (uterus), and finally she is guided to meet him in a Paris train station cafe where it is possible to hear the *departures* being announced. This film was perhaps my most evocative experience of twin loss.

GENERATIONAL PATTERNS

Australian psychiatrist Avril Earnshaw discovered that major events, such as illness, birth, miscarriage, death, divorce, and emigration, tend to be repeated through generations. She believes that our genes are "time-tagged" so that an important event may occur when the offspring reaches the same age at which a major event occurred for the same-sex parent, especially the birth of a sibling to the offspring and the offspring's birth. Since becoming acquainted with her work I always note any such synchronicities in the family history of my clients. (This information can be elicited with the questionnaire and genogram described in Appendix 1.) It is not infrequent that a child will be conceived on a mother's birthday, or on the day that a family member died, for example. Sometimes children in the same family have identical birthdays. Frequently, people will marry, divorce, or die at the same age as their same-sex parent—chronogenetics is a good party topic.

Being aware of these generational patterns, I took great care to avoid any big shifts in my life as I approached the age of forty, which was my mother's age when I was born. That was one of my more intuitive decisions, for something major did occur—she died. Since I already had learned that the death of the mother's mother is a deep tragedy for a baby in utero, I was relieved that I had not been pregnant during that year. I also separated from my husband at that time.

The context of my development has helped provide a framework for me to understand and change many patterns in my life, and to be more observant with my children of those old patterns which are proving recalcitrant!

PERSONAL INSIGHTS

I first left home at the age of sixteen, when I went to the United States as an exchange student from Australia. I shared the nine-month school year and mutual activities with the other exchange student—a male. On returning to Australia I explained this bond to my mentor. "But we shared everything— excursions, travel, social events—as the male/female exchange student pair—I could never again find such an ideal foundation for a relationship." I was stunned that he strongly disagreed, remarking that I could walk out right then and meet someone just as special in the elevator! I maintained that connection in the hope of an eventual union, hanging on as surviving twins always do, through long years of correspondence while I completed college. Members of my family teased me, accurately predicting that it "wouldn't work out" a concept which stirred my anguish at the thought of a repetition of my fetal drama. In keeping with my desire to get away, I eventually journeyed to the most densely-populated country in Europe (a crowded wombspace) and we became engaged. (Ironically, after we split, I learned that my ex-fiance's sister and only sibling was later killed in a plane crash.)

My impulse for as long as I can remember was "to get away." Because I always felt wrong, I felt pressured to do more, to prove myself, to be clever in compensation. I believed that I needed to carry burdens and looked for struggles. If things seemed easy in my life, I found ways to increase the load. At university, I felt it wasn't enough to be enrolled full time in physical therapy training; I took English literature to work toward a B.A. in addition. When I worked all day as a physical therapist, it didn't seem enough, so I took courses at night in Dutch, then Italian. (Interestingly, I chose language courses—expressing my uterine need to communicate. Of course, languages would help me when I got away.) Later, I studied full time for a B.A. degree while I developed my physical therapy practice; doing two jobs at once. I was only too happy to be the breadwinner when my husband wanted to go to business school in the United States. I had no ambitions of my own at all; now that I had got away from my home and country, I saw my role as helping things happen in my husband's life.

My placental experience had left me with a decisive feeling that I never wanted to be on the end of anyone else's lifeline again. I hated the times of my life when I was salaried; my choice is to be self-employed and ride out the highs and lows. I prefer to be independent and in control, and this has led to relationships with men who needed me to be self-supporting (or even providing support) because they were studying, burdened with punitive alimony and child-support payments, or else voluntarily chose not to work for remuneration. I was thus attempting to rescue my lost twin in a recreated environment of inadequate placental nourishment (money is a form of sustenance and nurture). Also, I have repeatedly found myself in relationships requiring uterine symbols of conveyance—commuting by train, car or plane for months or even years. Today, my husband works half the week almost 2 hours away from the family; a similar situation but the traveler is reversed. I also understand my resentment when Geoff left me for a summer with my two year old, to move into and paint an old house (womb) while he went out to Australia to build a new house for his sister. It was about a week after his return that Julia lost her finger—I sense a connnection with his circumcision which was a body amputation for him likewise happening shortly after the completion of his gestational house (term of pregnancy).

My relationship with Geoff brought up issues of implantation—attachment to the uterine wall. I felt that there had to be more beneath his surface, behind his "wall." I could continue to chip away at the buried treasure within him only for as long as I could see the end (the birth). The years dragged on and I felt increasingly constricted and internally confused until he agreed to a separation. My primal imprint was "even though this cord is bringing in nothing that I want and need, I have to stay attached for my own survival." Of course, my mind turned it around that *he* needed to stay attached to *me* for *his* survival, and I did hang on until he was ready to go.

It is not unrelated that Geoff's presentation prior to birth had been breech. The doctor turned him around and tied an "irritation pad" over him so he couldn't get into that position again. This was also a major irritation to his mother, a naturally nurturing woman, who as a result was unable to take a bath or shower for the rest of the pregnancy. No wonder Geoff had a hard time finding his niche—his rightful place in life—and often felt stuck. He also may have suffered an imprint of abandonment when, at the age of twelve months, he was taken away to live with a relative because his mother was erroneously diagnosed as having tuberculosis and sent to a sanitarium. Other children in the family teased him that she was dead, and indeed in the young child's mind separation from mother is equated with death. In his marriage it seems as if he found the same situation in which a woman would ultimately "abandon" him. Until then, our negative uterine experiences brought us together. We always enjoyed traveling in search of the perfect ocean beach—a primal need we both shared to find oceanic bliss, to sink into the support of soft but supportive sand, and to feel the nurturing warmth from the radiant sun. I agree with Harriet Goldhor Lerner, author of *The Dance of Anger* and *The Dance of Intimacy*, that the very qualities that make couples angry with each other are the ones that attracted them together in the first place. I married my lost twin!

As a result of my prenatal dynamics I have been committed to completing a job, keeping to my word; I would rather get something over and done with than postpone it. This is because I feel sure that, at the end, there will be "more"—especially emotional contact.

Significantly, during some physical construction we did for a business venture, and at the same time that Geoff's infertility was discovered, I was diagnosed with thoracic outlet syndrome. Although I did not have the extra ribs in my neck that cause this nerve compression, I had surgery to remove the first ribs and associated fibrous bands that had the same effect (weakness and wasting of small muscles in my hands). The muscles involved are clearly marked on Johnsen's chart of prefunctional muscles, and the hypotonia is a result of prenatal freezing. The immobilization of my arms in my crib further compounded that imprint.

While my shoulders only ached occasionally, I see the muscle damage and as a direct result of trying to "shoulder" everything. I now appreciate what Bernie Siegel means when he says it is the sick person who always says yes to requests from friends. The ability to say no is essential for a healthy immune system, found in people who have developed enough intelligent self-interest to meet their own needs first.

PROFESSIONAL INSIGHTS

In addition to these personal connections that I made with regard to my relationships, facets of my professional work seemed to fall into place. I am convinced that the assumptions I made during the *first few weeks* of my embryonic existence were the basis of all my career choices. I have always been more drawn to pregnancy and conception (where, of course, I needed to do my own healing) rather than birth (which for me was quick, easy, and without any outside intervention).

Because my mother was on bed rest when she carried me, I later pioneered prenatal exercise via books, videos, lectures, and workshops. My existential ambivalence was expressed in not wanting to breathe, and in my professional work I have always spoken out against "controlled breathing"—the artificial respiratory patterns taught to pregnant women as a "distraction" for use during labor, and the forced breath-holding prior to birth. I questioned these practices first in *Essential Exercises for the Childbearing Year*, long before I knew about primal memory. In this book, I simply explained the normal physiology of breathing and muscle action in pregnancy, birth, and postpartum, just as in *Having Twins* I reassured expectant mothers of multiples to eat for two, keep exercising, bond with the babies, and search for providers who support natural childbirth.

The idea that laboring women should simply breathe as they wish continues to be met with enormous resistance from maternity-care providers. And I continue to put forth Graham's insight that this resistance is related to their birth anxiety. What else could it be, when the physiological arguments are entirely sound and have been documented scientifically for decades?

My mother, fortunately, was not forced to pant like a small dog, nor would she have had time, since I arrived in less than ten minutes. My rapid birth, however, ruined my mother's pelvic floor muscles and she later had extensive surgery, first "general repairs" and then a hysterectomy for prolapse of her uterus. As a result I have been a strong advocate of pelvic floor exercises—preventively and therapeutically—for over twenty years.

All of these gestational experiences led me to found the Obstetrics and Gynecology Section of the American Physical Therapy Association and the Maternal and Child Health Center in Cambridge. It was my dream to create a venue for pregnant women to gather *because* they are pregnant; in the world today most of them carry on *in spite of* being pregnant, often an unfortunate denial that is a career imperative.

I directed that center for eleven years, although I very much wanted to hand it over after *nine* years, when I was pregnant with my son, and especially by the *ninth* month. Significantly, during the last two years that I directed the center, I expended a lot of time and energy looking for a new location. Although for many reasons that was quite legitimate—we had grown and the space was dilapidated—it was still a primal "house" issue for me. It became progressively more difficult for me to go there—physically to go up stairwells and corridor (tubes) into the old womb. I needed to be born into a new place if I were to stay in charge. But I already had our newly constructed lakeside house and clinic a hundred miles away. Symbolically, at my farewell party an old telephone cord was produced and the cord cut by my successors. I understood this primal ritual in the light of their claim that I was too "radical," (from the Latin, *radix*, meaning root.) To connect with roots is threatening—severance is a logical reaction. Anthropologically, placental rituals reduce anxiety when there is a transition into the unknown with its dual aspects of power and danger.

Thus in 1990 I was freed to be reborn into new roles and ventures, in an ideal esthetic environment for writing, teaching, and seeing clients. I wanted more time to think creatively about pre- and perinatal issues, especially since an increasing number of people came to me with physical and psychological problems that originated at birth and before.

CHAPTER ELEVEN

Birth Burdens and Unkind Cuts

Birth—What futility to believe that so great a
cataclysm will not leave its mark.
Its traces are everywhere, in the skin, in the bones,
in the stomach, in the back
In all our human folly
In our madness, our tortures, our prisons
In legends, epics, myths
In the Scriptures.

— FREDERICK LEBOYER

We have seen that normal births can be stressful for the baby who enters the world headfirst. The experience of being born differently from the usual head-down way, in breech presentation, or by Cesarean section is explored next. And the perinatal events of cutting the cord (for all babies) and cutting the foreskin (for unfortunate male infants) also have potential long-term effects that I examine in this chapter.

BREECH PRESENTATION

Mothers of breech babies, Cheek found, usually were not happy at news of pregnancy or else they became distressed for some reason at the end of their pregnancy. Their emotional state made it difficult for the baby to overcome the uterine tension and present with his head.

Mechanical factors may also cause a baby to present with the bottom half of his body. He is able to change position until about the thirty-second week of pregnancy. Since the uterus is egg-shaped, with less space at the bottom, if the baby flexes his knees he will assume a head-down position, whereas if he extends them he will fit better as a breech. Backache in the mother and misalignment of her spine can also influence her baby's options.

Doctors sometimes attempt to turn the baby head down (external version). This doesn't always work and second attempts can be made, usually in the hospital with tocolytic drugs to relax the uterus. Cheek found that by using language instead of version, if the pregnancy was at least three weeks before term, his success rate was 60 percent. He now recommends that if the fetus cannot be persuaded to turn we should respect his choice in assuming that position. Liley said likewise, that the "fetus knows better than the obstetrician how he'll be most comfortable." But with a Cesarean almost guaranteed by today's fearful obstetricians I believe version should always be attempted. Obstetrician Leo Sorger has applied the principles of haptonomy, and his success rate with versions has increased since he began guiding the mother to relax her uterus and make contact with the baby during the procedure. If version doesn't succeed, we both recommend a breech delivery in the absence of complications.

Although some breech babies deliver spontaneously (especially in the squatting position), others need to be extracted. Since the head is the last part to be delivered, and the arms may be over the head, experience and skill are required. Some breeches will put their arms out to the side, gesturing that they don't want to slide down into the pelvis, usually with a valid reason—such as a short cord.

I remember a woman who didn't want her baby turned: "I was born breech, so was my mother and my grandmother. This is the way we come out in our family!" she said. Breeches who resist version, according to Graham, want the struggle. The influence of distortion and feeling wrong, however, may lead them to feel in later life that others are always trying to turn them or "their opinion" around. A mother told me how her twins, both born breech, always go down a slide in birth order. Both insist "that's the way it is supposed to be."

Jeannine Parvati Baker, a midwife, writer, and lecturer in

the pre- and perinatal field, has experienced six births and loved birthing her breech twin, claiming that "somehow it felt that this was the way it should be."

I observed in Graham's clinic that the proportion of adults who were of breech presentation was much higher than the average 3 percent in the general population. Obviously, it is a more difficult way to be born, and there are often significant prenatal factors that motivate the individual to seek regression therapy.

RESOLUTION OF RESIDUAL EFFECTS
OF TRAUMATIC BREECH BIRTH

Penny had a long history of chronic functional weakness on her left side. Despite months of physical therapy, shortening and rotation persisted at her left hip. During the treatment sessions, where her arms would be stretched over her head, Penny would recall an attempted rape by her great-uncle at age five. When her left leg was exercised, Penny felt cold in the lower half of her body but the trunk and area above her waist felt warm. Her therapist intuited that she had been born breech. Penny felt there was something deep inside causing her problems. She knew intuitively that the surgery that her family and doctor kept encouraging her to undergo would not solve the problem, so she came to see if I could help.

On the floor, her initial bodily sensations were of being twisted, "wound up tightly like yarn on a spool," starting with a "knot" and going up through her back, the pain ending with a feeling of pressure in her head. Penny also re-experienced her foot "caught on something" as the hip and knee were maximally flexed, until the foot "popped free." She had told me earlier that her predominant feeling in life was that her head was separated from the rest of her body.

She returned later that evening and explored feelings in her throat and head. She described how she had lost the ability to elevate her arms, and when this was done passively in physical therapy, she recalled her great-uncle's attack when he held her arms over her head and said "If you scream, I'll kill you." Penny had always been plagued with laryngitis and headaches, and had great difficulty making sound during therapy.

For three sessions she repeated the twisting to the right, and her movements were always in the direction of her feet, also consistent with a breech delivery. I suggested that "the band, hooking on . . . if only I could just get it to snap off" could be the obstetrician's fingers, grabbing her leg in the groin to both rotate the pelvis and bring it down. She responded with instant recognition. It was clear to me at that time that he rotated her in the wrong direction, with considerable force distracting her hip joint. Since her head was trapped higher up on the pelvic brim, this had the effect of also forcing her head and neck back, and tightening the "smooth rope" around her neck. So only by flexing and pulling "in" could she relieve the pain and pressure of being strangled and suffocated by the cord around her neck. No wonder this set up a lifetime pattern of her head and body pulling in opposite directions.

Penny's experience led me to an insight regarding a potential problem with all breeches. Since head extension is the usual feature of sperm memory, and in the usual presentations the head is mechanically flexed by the shape of the pelvis, the breech whose head prior to birth is floating in the top of the uterus has to make a choice between flexion and extension. Extension is to get trapped. Powerful, painful memories of sperm penetration could easily trigger the same pattern of extension, which will delay or prevent the birth, something Penny also relived. Subsequently, she completely and spontaneously re-birthed herself, with the movement beginning with her head for the first time in full flexion, and also for the first time rotating in the correct direction. As she moved feet first past the resistance I provided, she gave a visible sigh of joy and relief, and expressed how wonderful that first breath of air felt. I have checked with this patient for several years now and she has had no relapse of her hip problems: a dramatic resolution.

Very few obstetricians take on the risk of a breech delivery in today's medicolegal climate. However, during breech births manual pressure on the baby at the top of the uterus is commonly done. It must be done with great awareness so that the head is flexed; indeed the baby could also be asked to flex his head with some gentle guidance.

CESAREAN SECTION

Birth is such a powerful imprint that it is difficult for some women who have not been born vaginally to give birth in this way. Cesarean birth is thus a marker in a woman's history. She and her health-care providers need to be aware that blocks in labor may arise, and the issues are ideally resolved beforehand. Cesarean-born adults may not want to perpetuate their experience of birth and the life scripts that often follow. Women are often afraid to become pregnant and run the risk of having the belly cut open.

There are two kinds of Cesareans: one is an emergency after labor has begun, and the other is scheduled (often for convenience) and is known as a nonlabor Cesarean. Each type sets up different dynamics. A period of labor produces hormonal changes and physical stimuli that physiologically ready the baby's systems for birth. This preparation is missing in the nonlabor situation, where the baby is plucked out of the womb.

Although the obvious physical sensations of vaginal delivery are missing, there may nevertheless be much pulling and tugging by the obstetricians to dislodge a wedged breech or head. Accidental injuries with the scalpels may occur. Suctioning is more likely because the amniotic fluid is not squeezed out of the chest, as in a vaginal delivery. The baby may experience lack of oxygen as he is lifted up above his blood supply, and he is usually separated from his mother for twenty-four hours of "observation."

In *The Healing Power of Birth*, Rima Beth Star (Cunningham) describes how the doctor had nicked her ear during her Cesarean delivery. She was aware that the nurses and doctor were terrified that they had hurt her and that she might die. Her personal law became: "people who love me, hurt me."

As I began to understand these experiences, my life began to make more sense. I understood the connection between physical pain and love. I understood why I had dreamed about knives, why I was not as close to people as I wanted to be, why I put a child between myself and others. These were issues which controlled my life because I had never examined the decision I made. Yet I operated as though these decisions were laws handed down to me, as though I had no choice in the matter. . . . It was very liberating to discover that I had created these "laws" myself, and that I could recreate my life. I could now make new laws about life and, in doing so, improve my relationships. In fact, when my perspective of the past changed, the present seemed to change as well.

After an unsatisfactory first birth experience with forceps, Rima pursued regression experiences, which allowed her to resolve her birth issues to the extent that she subsequently had three water births at home. This is all the more amazing considering that her first child drowned in a friend's pool.

Jane English described her regression experiences in *Different Doorway: Adventures of a Cesarean Born*. She speculated that people delivered surgically have a different way of being in the world—that is, particularly regarding time and space—than those who "pushed through" the vagina. Her personal journey recounts her coming to terms with issues she believes may be characteristic for a nonlabor Cesarean, such as helplessness, boundaries, victimization, and separation. There is a difference between Cesareans and the vaginally born in their position on the continuum between total separation and total oneness, according to English, who felt that much of her fighting with the world was over boundaries. "So many people say I demand too much. I have learned I am supposed to have boundaries so I continually test where they are."

Birth influences the dynamics of relationships, and there are special dimensions in those who were surgically delivered. Cesarean babies may better tolerate great pressure, sudden change, and lack of definition. A rapid entry into the world gives a different imprint from the ebb and flow of labor contractions for the vaginally born. English wrote: "I tend to be direct, all or nothing, like an arrow." She pointed out that Cesarean birth is not limited in time to the removal of the baby from the mother, but continues for years. "That Cesareans appear 'unborn' is one manifestation of this; their births are still in process." When a birth doesn't happen naturally, the baby doesn't feel responsible for it. This may set up a need to find someone who constantly will "give birth" to them, even if it requires being "torn out of comfortable situations." That dependence of the Cesarean born is also shared to some degree by those delivered by instruments.

Cesareans tend not to know how to push through barriers and break out of structures; their birth script is often to look for a savior because that is what happened during birth. "I want to learn about pushing through," wrote English, but it has to be without the vaginally born person's belief that if they *don't* push through they will die. For me it is just the opposite. I fear that if I *do* push I might die."

In a Cesarean birth, the baby suddenly leaves the envelope of his mother's energy. Always an abrupt transition, it can also be an emergency operation with much fear and tension. As a result, Cesarean-born adults may tend "to wait for everything to disappear, especially comfort," which causes feelings of mistrust and insecurity to arise. As English wrote: "I notice that I did not want to know what I wanted in the world because I was afraid that it would be taken away from me if I got it. I wasn't prepared for letting go of my mother that fast."

Another Cesarean-born adult agreed:

I definitely know that at birth I thought they were killing me. I remember distinctly the fear and panic. . . . Then I thought they had killed my mother. Cesareans have a tendency to be angry, helpless and needy, although this may not be obvious. . . . If I go into a room, the people to whom I respond most, I often find out, are Cesarean.

If there is no period of contractions before the operation, doctors and nurses, rather than mothers, "labor" with a Cesarean baby. General anesthesia (which is rare today) has been experienced as poisoning, nausea, hot and cold, being alone and being attached, fear of leaving the body, quietly dying, and "feeling sad at having to abandon form." The incision came as a shock, a rape, "shuddering" to English because she was still drugged and unable to resist. The first touch is an "electrical awakening," a mixture of pleasure and pain, but it lacks the wholeness, integrity, and coherence of the physical sensations of total body stimulation in the vagina. English feels that the first greeting would be potentially positive if Cesarean babies were handled with more awareness and sensitivity. It has been suggested that delivering the baby within intact membranes would ease the transition as well as filter the bright light and sounds and buffer the change in temperature and pressure.

Cutting the cord is felt as a "death, defeat, total loss of support, tension in belly." English experienced the stimulation to start breathing and clear the lungs as "being attacked, murderous anger, fighting my own breathing coming as yet another strange, scary sensation, orgiastic experience of energy in the body." Even though delivery is complete, she pointed out that this experience is still very much part of birth: "The bond with my mother was broken. I bonded with him [the doctor] and then felt totally shattered when he, too, left me. I think consciously I have been reliving this pattern with men ever since."

While separation happens in a normal birth (a senseless and regrettable routine that is slowly dying out), this is worse after a Cesarean birth because mother and baby need each other even more. English explained that grief is a natural process after the separation of two beings who have been as one. This separation requires a radical readjustment:

> I was prevented by the anesthesia from fully mourning. I think of the great raw place in myself I feel in myself. It may have no psychological content and may be at this cellular level, the tearing apart of two beings. I have projected it onto the surgery, onto learning to breathe, onto people, onto the whole world. At its root, it is a psychic wound.

There is much room for improvement in Cesarean birth. The nurses and doctors must realize that in a nonlabor Cesarean the baby's first touch experience—suctioning and wiping—must be done gently, as a form of emotional and spiritual labor. In a way *they* are the ones giving birth; they are "breaking into" the mother to deliver the baby, and this contrasts with the "pushing out" of vaginal birth.

The Cesarean baby breathes out of fear; he is forced into it rather than experiences it as a choice, a natural sequence. Sometimes the baby breathes by tuning into the doctor's breathing and merging with him emotionally. The mother doesn't feel as if she has given birth, and this feeling is accentuated by the separation. Cesarean babies must remain with their mothers unless there is sufficient medical emergency to justify an interruption of the bonding.

In English's second book, *Cesarean Born*, she created a map that will help Cesarean people and show, by contrast, the vaginal birth map. She concluded: "We have to go deeper to find our common human experience. Going deeper is a step in the direction of experiencing the awareness of unity or oneness." If the birth experience is the paradigm for change, then the Cesarean-born will have a different paradigm for what change is and how it happens. Cesareans' unfamiliarity with boundaries may give them access to higher consciousness without having to push through. English claimed that a positive advantage of Cesarean birth is an "ideal structure for allowing something new to come through into the world. It sets aside deep patterns that have been common to all human culture."

Many therapists today help children and mothers cope with Cesarean birth, especially when the mother feels that it was an unnecessary intervention. Dowling found the story of Little Red Riding Hood "perfectly designed for the therapeutic handling of the birth trauma in children." The girl—little, red, and with her head covered (in a caul)—returns to the womb that already contains her grandmother (the placenta). Instead of dying, she is rescued when the wolf's belly is cut open.

Graham often closes his workshops with healing circles— for example, all those who were born by Cesarean gather in the outer circle, around an inner circle of those who gave birth by Cesarean. These pairs have the opportunity to express feelings about their respective experiences and share comfort and support.

THE UNTOLD SIGNIFICANCE OF THE UMBILICAL CORD

Using ultrasound, the unborn baby has been seen grasping the cord at nine weeks. It is a significant connection for him to his periphery—his placenta and his mother. Lake emphasized the influence of chronic negative umbilical affect on the unborn baby; in a toxic womb "longing can turn to loathing" and birth is an escape. Feeding or sucking and umbilical exchange are closely related; thumbsucking is viewed as a substitute for an inadequate cord. Sucking by the fetus has been said to bring about contractions of his abdominal muscles, which enable the baby to exert some sense of control over what is going in and out of his navel.

Umbilical artery flow becomes the root for later experiences of excretion, according to Mott. The fetus feels drawn into the placenta, he journeys forth, and gains a primary sense of orientation, a structure of space and time. The "single straight aggressive thrust" from the placenta also restores. The venous flow is a primary act of ingestion, the root for later experiences of eating and drinking. The placenta thus has ambivalent roles as receptacle for excretion and an instrument of food. It is hollow and helpless, yet solid and aggressive.

I can recall one baby who was so entangled in his cord that it was like string around a package. This infant survived an unplanned conception, an ambivalent gestation (several appointments for an abortion were made and canceled), and was finally delivered by emergency Cesarean. The child had very delayed control of his excretory functions and is a "very poor eater" even into his school years.

Psychiatrist John Diamond, author of *The Body Doesn't Lie* and *Behavioral Kinesiology*, has made the umbilicus the keystone of his work with muscle testing to discover unconscious thoughts and motivations, having noted that all the acupuncture meridians are concentrated around the umbilicus.

SEVERING THE CORD— CUTTING THE CONNECTION

Fodor felt that Freudians "shrunk from admitting the trauma of the cutting the cord" because it would reflect on Freud that he had missed something so important. Laing observed that the cord and placenta can take on phantom limb-like phenomena, in which people still feel the pain, for example, of an amputated limb. "I am impressed," he wrote, "by the fact that "I" was once placenta, umbilical cord, and fetus. . . . all cellularly, biologically, physically, *genetically, me*."

Postpartum, an umbilical crisis can arise when the cord is cut. Although the baby does not feel the pain of the cutting, he may be suddenly forced to breathe or suffocate. Grof wrote of "a sharp pain in the navel, loss of breath, fear of death and castration." Cutting the cord too soon, together with separating the baby from the mother, is a double injury. One doesn't have to be a Freudian to speculate about castration fears and to realize that certainly some sadomasochism results from primal imprints—wanting to be tied up, having to struggle in pain, and reproducing other cord dramas. Some unfortunate people who are born with the cord around the neck commit suicide by strangulation.

A significant feeling of loss and detachment may be experienced on the psychological level. Leslie Feher described in *The Psychology of Birth* a "natal therapy" whereby participants actually wear a fake umbilical cord. It has been suggested that recognition of the man having more of the symbolic umbilicus left after birth than a woman may play a role in male chauvinism. Perhaps that is why men persist in the strange custom of wearing neckties.

Many children will cling to a doll, soft toy, or an old blanket, especially at night. Dowling pointed out that these "transitional objects" represent the placenta. Such objects are frequently associated with oral (such as thumbsucking) or anal behavior (when the object becomes dirty and smelly). This is important for its symbolic function as an organ of excretion, and if it is washed the child may search again for a suitable representation of placental projections.

The cord is also considered an object of security. That first loss, if not handled sensitively, will reverberate through other losses in later life. My daughter Julia, who lost her left index finger at age two and a half, subsequently suffered intermittent "tummyaches" that were localized at her navel. (Apley's rule, developed by an astute physician, stated: "The further the site of the pain from the umbilicus the more likely it is to be organic." Therefore, precise umbilical pain can be assumed to be primal in origin.) Indeed, there were never clinical signs of intestinal dysfunction.

When Graham learned that Julia's cord had been cut immediately after birth, he made the connection that the sight of her missing finger brought back the trauma of the sudden loss of her cord. This diagnosis has been confirmed on several occasions when other children have observed Julia's missing finger and immediately complained of pain in *their* navels! In each case, the mother verified that the cord was cut before it stopped pulsing. As Julia grew older, these tummyaches became less frequent and disappeared, but it was helpful to all of us that after her session with Graham she was able to refer to the real issue and could call it her "cord pain."

Boadella warned that if the cord is cut too soon, the infant will experience a circulatory and a respiratory shock, a wash-back effect from blood that would have returned to mother, putting stress on the heart and depriving the baby of oxygen and red blood cells. At the same time the baby needs to take in oxygen all at once in his newly expanded lungs, and this is achieved naturally if the cord is allowed to wither as it is exposed to air. The jelly around the blood vessels congeals, gradually halting the flow of blood and permitting a smooth transition.

Even when all pulsing in the cord has ceased, the time may not be right to sever it. Parents should consult the newborn, and allow plenty of time for him to release this genetically identical "partner" and long-time intimate companion. Physiologically, the placenta still supplies oxygen after delivery, so that the baby has time to adjust to using his lungs. How we breathe at birth determines how we will breathe for the rest of our life, warned LeBoyer. Some home birthers, such as Jeannine Parvati Baker, actually leave the placenta attached to the baby (a "lotus birth") until the cord naturally drops off a few days later.

My son Carsten was born underwater. The cord usually pulsates longer when submerged because it is not exposed to air. About forty minutes after birth we were ready to cut the cord, but Carsten stopped nursing and started to wail. We waited until he seemed ready, and he remained calm when his cord was tied and then cut. We took several photos of the placenta before burying it in the garden (a symbolic rebirth) under a now-thriving Colorado blue spruce. In many cultures, the placenta is afforded this kind of respect, but in modern hospitals the parents may never see the placenta, which is discarded.

CIRCUMCISION

My anguish over Julia's loss of a finger has fueled the energy I put into the anticircumcision movement. Having watched my child suffer the loss of a body part, I will never understand why and how could anyone *choose* to remove a healthy body part, and against the vociferous protests of the victim.

Cutting genitals is culturally accepted in the United States. Episiotomies are cut to enlarge the vagina for birth, and almost half of baby boys are circumcised in the United States—from habit, ignorance, and religion.

In the United States non-Orthodox Jews and Moslems as well as the majority of Americans have been submitting their infants to circumcision for generations. Routine neonatal circumcision is done soon after birth, so I have included it as a perinatal trauma. Newborns vividly remember pain and deeply resent interference with their bodily integrity without their knowledge and consent. There are now several videotapes available showing this barbaric act as well as many studies documenting increased crying, heart rates, adrenalin levels, and sleep disturbances. If parents could identify and empathize with their unborn child, they would never agree to this perverse practice. Health insurance in some states no longer covers this totally unnecessary and harmful surgery.

Many of Graham's clients have relived the agony of circumcision, done (and continues to be done) *without* anesthesia. David Chamberlain, in an article "Babies Remember Pain," quotes one of his clients:

There's a sensation I've never experienced before. It's in my back, being drawn up, pulled in. I don't know where I am but I feel like my shoulder blades are not resting comfortably and my shoulders are pushing down. I can't bend them. I'm on something hard and cold! I feel myself arching. It's cold! I feel my whole body arching now. I don't know what's going on. I hear babies crying and I'm crying too. I don't know why. Oh! They are pulling on my penis and I'm feeling some pain. It hurts there; I'm not sure why. There's a white robe: it's a doctor. They are holding my legs down and my back is arched. They are cutting my penis and it hurts. It hurts! I feel my penis being pulled. I feel sharp points there. I'm hurting and my back is tight. Someone picks me up and holds me. I can't relax. I am stiff. My penis hurts; it burns. It hurts and I can't relax. Even when I'm bundled up I can't relax. It takes a long time to relax. . . . I'm tired now. I cried hard. I'm all cried out. I'm trying to go to sleep.

While Jews account for less than 2 percent of the circumcisions done in the United States, many of them are speaking out against the ritual and devising a celebration without mutilation. If these inspiring activists can say no to such a cultural and religious imperative, there is hope for change in any human endeavor.

For nearly two decades I have directed my attention toward enhancing natural childbirth practices. Ironically, many pioneers in Cesarean prevention and other aspects of the movement went right on to circumcise their own sons, or to sit on the fence when the procedure was discussed in childbirth class. Some parents who engage in prenatal bonding, and have home births and LeBoyer baths, nevertheless subject their infant to this unnecessary removal of a sexually important body part. Some natural childbirth enthusiasts wax lyrical about "primitive birth," when often the young girls will be subject to an even grosser form of genital mutilation. (Primarily in Africa, over 100 million females have had their clitoris and/or labia excised.)

Physicians who are sworn to "above all, do no harm" have been the major stumbling block toward reform in the United States. Not only do they promote circumcision (for which they get paid) but they also misinform on a large scale the wise and caring parents who wish to keep their sons intact.

The time has come to honor, respect, and protect the new life we are privileged to bring into this uncertain world. We cannot always prevent negative prenatal imprints or even a traumatic birth experience. But we can take care not to add insult to injury with genital mutilation.

CHAPTER TWELVE

Double Realities: Adoption and Twins

Civilisation will commence on the day when the well-being of the newborn baby will prevail over any other consideration.
—WILHELM REICH

A baby's experience of adoption or twinship is one of "double realities—two mothers in the case of adoption and two babies in the case of twins. With adoption and the loss of a twin, death is the divider, and although it is a symbolic death when a baby is relinquished by his or her mother, the effect is the same. Pre- and perinatal memories of these events have revealed their profound impact, and call for much greater sensitivity and awareness on the part of both professionals and parents in these situations.

ADOPTION

Adoption has been called the "primal wound." Regardless of how much love and devotion is shown by the adopting parents or other primary caregivers, and even if the adoptee later accepts the reasons for the relinquishment, the baby inside always feels abandoned. No foster parents and institutions, however exemplary, can enter into the same psychic bond that the prenatal community of life and immediate postnatal maternal care establish. In the biological mother, the maternal physiological functions are merged with her emotions, and this is a necessary foundation for security, self-esteem, and a satisfying mother-child relationship. Winnicott's concept of primary maternal preoccupation explains how a mother can identify with her infant, and thus by feeling herself in his or her place, meet her infant's needs. A mother's ability to give her baby a secure start in life emotionally is based on this powerful feeling. This process, which is disrupted by adoption, is also often impaired in premature birth. Thus "preemies" and adoptees both have difficulty in feeling ready to start life outside the womb and to trust the continuity of a secure existence.

This is not to say that adoption does not serve a useful purpose; clearly, family life is better than an orphanage or a rejecting mother. But adoption cannot match the ideal continuity of mutually affective pre- and perinatal relationships, and the bonds that develop organically. Separation from the birth mother is a source of pain and anxiety that violates feelings of safety and security; both mother and baby feel grief. Evolution planned for a sequence of events around birth, which are triggered hormonally as well as emotionally.

Adoption counselor Nancy Verrier points out that there are three ways of entering a family: birth, adoption, and marriage. Only marriage implies choice on the part of the individual, but with birth he or she has an inherent biological right to be there. In the case of adoption there is neither choice nor inalienable right to help the relationship. As a matter of fact, says Verrier, "adoption begins with failure": failure on the part of the birth parents to be willing or able to take care of their child, and failure on the part of the adoptive parents (in most cases) to be able to conceive.

Bonding with the adoptive mother is a greater challenge when it has been completely lacking in the birth mother. French psychologist Paul Madaule has used the "electronic ear," a device developed by Dr. Alfred Tomatis to screen out the high frequencies in the adoptive mother's voice so that it sounds as it would from inside the uterus. This apparently helps to decrease the impact of the "rejection complex" and facilitate attachment to the adoptive mother.

The impact of birth rejection paradoxically leads the adoptee to seek rejection in later life as a way of searching for love. His rage against the biological mother may be directed, sometimes relentlessly, against the adoptive mother. Some children withdraw and others test all the limits, as if to say, "How badly do I have to behave for you to prove you will never withdraw your love for me?" Children who don't cause trouble may seem untroubled, but this may not be true—simply that the baby inside "has died." Adoptees must be given a safe space to explore their primal wound and express their feelings.

Adoptees frequently state that they don't feel "real," which dates back from their earliest beginnings inside a mother who was emotionally absent during an unplanned and unwanted pregnancy. The trauma begins well before relinquishment, usually at implantation, which is the first contact the fertilized egg has with its mother. Adoptees, like others who develop in a hostile uterine environment, can only feel "real" if they feel pain, because that was their primary experience at the beginning of their existence. To be alive is to be in pain, to connect is to experience rejection. Such an engram can lead to much self-destructive activity in later life.

The feeling of isolation and alienation is reinforced if the birth mother never holds her infant. In fact, the touching, the need to feel the mother's skin, is very important in the establishment of "I" and "the other," a sense of boundaries that is crucial to self-identity. Many adoptees and their birth mothers later express deep regret at never seeing or *touching* each other. Adoptees who relive their birth often cry out in agony for "just a moment of touch," never having felt body contact from their mother "on the outside." This primal loss can give rise to a lifelong feeling of deprivation.

Mott emphasized that the fetal skin is part of the experience of being: the fetus does not "have" a skin, he "is" his skin. This is the foundation of haptonomy, wherein skin reflexes and perceptions can be altered by affective contact.

When I was a student at a maternity hospital in Australia, the doctor would say "F.A." (For Adoption) and pass the baby behind his back, where the waiting hands of the nurse would whisk it away. The unfortunate mother never had one glimpse of the child she carried for nine months. Fortunately, social pressure and legislation has put a stop to this dehumanizing practice, and the rights of the birth mother are now recognized and protected.

Verny stated that adopted children start life with a handicap—the sense of rejection by their own mothers, however devoted the adoptive parents may be. An adoptee's disturbed sense of self shows in a sense of mistrust, depression, anxiety, and difficulties in relationships. I know of an adoptee who in graduate school revealed that he could never ring the doorbell of someone he had come to visit without first going around to look in all the windows. (The window being a symbol of the birth canal, it is understandable that he wanted to check out who was on the other side.) From 30 to 40 percent of children found in special schools, mental health facilities, and residential treatment centers are adopted. As I write this, it came to my attention that at the Yale Juvenile Psychiatric Institute, the number of adoptees is 60 percent. Adoptees have more problems in school, socially as well as academically, and have a higher incidence of running away from home, juvenile delinquency, and sexual promiscuity. A female adoptee may fall into her mother's pattern and punish herself for hating her by becoming the mother of a child herself, so that the pattern of generational pain is repeated.

Also, adoptees are more likely to engage in criminal activity than other members of the public. Son of Sam, the Boston Strangler, and the L.A. Strangler were all adoptees. Son of Sam was a forceps baby who put a gun to his victims' temples, and the other two killers had experienced the cord around their neck at birth and symbolically repeated the same strangulation trauma on their victims.

The adoption system with its closed records and secrecy causes adoptees to feel "not born"; indeed, adoptees have traditionally been issued a second birth certificate as if by somehow rewriting names and facts a personal reality can be changed. Fortunately there is a trend today toward open and cooperative adoption. It is ideal if both parties can meet each other, but if not, adequate, accessible records must be kept that protect the rights of the child to know his or her truth. The battle to open the closed records still rages; judges deny adoptees access to their most important personal data, even in illness and old age. At this time only seven states allow adopted adults to find out who they are.

While both adoptees and birth mothers feel that their past is a total blank, with the facts locked away in sealed records and a false birth certificate, nevertheless everything is recorded organically. It is just a matter of accessing these unconscious memories. Understandably, adoptees are often reluctant to relive the pain of their pre- and perinatal period. I recently heard a sad story of a woman who had decided to give up her baby. She lied about her due date, fiddled with the fetal monitor to cause false "contractions," and begged for a Cesarean, all to get rid of the baby as early as possible. The adoptive family may never learn the extent of her rejection, but unfortunately, such imprints will program that baby's behavior for life.

As if the experience of adoption were not traumatic enough, most adoptees, like offspring from donor insemination, have been set back with deception as well. That is, they were brought up as the social parents' biological child without ever learning the truth of their origins. One small step in adoption reform has been the recognition that deception backfires profoundly; indeed, it is often viewed by the adoptee as worse than the relinquishment. Adoptees can feel compassion for their mother, whose circumstances usually forced her into giving her baby up without any choice. In contrast, they often feel nothing but outrage toward the social parents, who for their own protection deliberately chose to lie to their child. Today, adoptive parents are obliged to tell the child the truth as a prerequisite for acceptance by agencies. Unfortunately, this standard does not apply in the case of children conceived with donor sperm or eggs; the lesson of adoption deception has not yet been learned by practitioners of assisted conceptions. (For further discussion on this topic, see my book *Having Your Baby By Donor Insemination*.)

It is also important to support the adoptee in the search for his or her birth parents, however threatening this may be to the adoptive family. I encourage all adoptees who have symptoms of dysfunction or disease in their life, or general unhappiness, to explore regression as a way to fill in the missing pieces. Sometimes adoptees profess that they have no interest in knowing their past, but this is often denial of the early pain. Their motivation changes when they have their own children or undergo some life crisis. It *is* possible for a child to love more than one set of parents, just as parents can love more than one child. Invariably, the relationship with the adoptive parents improves after the search. In fact, some adoptees move beyond the pain of their mother's relinquishment and realize a deeper personal purpose. They believe that certain spirits arrive at their parental destination in this life only via adoption.

ADOPTION RELIVED

Helga was undergoing therapy with Graham, because of her need to "explore a void" she had been feeling. Unaware at age twenty-eight that she was an adoptee, she experienced a glass dome coming around her when Graham said he had information about her of which she was not aware. On learning this, Helga went into acute shock and rejected her mother. She felt deeply deceived and depressed after a Catholic upbringing emphasizing truthfulness. She actually lost muscle power in her left arm and leg, which CAT scans showed were normal. Helga felt shame at the knowledge of her adoption and blotches on her skin emerged. She knew she was desperately wanted by her adoptive parents, but she also felt that they were "hollow" and she had to somehow "fill them up," to take care of their emptiness and to make them feel special. As a result of healing her issues, Helga is now a therapist helping other adoptees to regress and resolve their primal wounds.

In another case, a woman connected her commitment to feminism with her adoption experience:

I remember the doctor rotating me to get me out. I was reluctant to let go of my mother, who was relinquishing me for adoption. The male doctor hurried my birth and I felt battered. Although I felt weary, that I made it, and made it as a woman, was a very powerful feeling.

Carol was not adopted, but her father left before she was born:

I recall being the happy sperm till I was obstructed. I tried to get around the block—it was crystal clear [the zona pellucida is a structureless membrane] she was angry. I really wanted to get through. Finally I did. I felt a great achievement until I realized it was a mistake and I wanted to get out. The egg pretended I wasn't there, with much sideways movement.

I had one beautiful memory of cell division, to African drum music. I felt myself dividing in two. It was the best experience I ever had. I felt so clear, so light, that I could spin through the room. I rolled around and people whom I touched said I was light.

In my adult life I have often felt blocked off and not heard in relationships. I took on my mother's fear of men by choosing schools of all girls and a female profession like nursing. I recognized that I needed to express myself in a way that doesn't feel blocked or unheard. This has been better since I have met my birth father. I feel more balance now. I trust my intuition and no longer feel hollow inside. After finally meeting my father, I felt like a spotlight shone on a huge dark area, above which there was a ladder going up and now I can reach the ladder.

The ladder, as we saw in Chapter 4, symbolizes the birth canal; for Carol, connecting with her paternal origins was a symbolic rebirth.

TWINS

Alessandra Piontelli has studied twins under ultrasound and confirmed that they interact in myriad ways clearly expressing their own identity and responding in different ways to their respective positions in the uterus. She points out that myths, legends and popular beliefs about twins attribute a "much more lively and adult life" to them than to singletons, who continue to be seen to some extent as "more passive, amorphous and little differentiated creatures, as if the fact of sharing the nine months of the pregnancy gave twins some kind of special attributes."

Conception, implantation, and birth present survival issues that are more of a challenge to twins than to singletons. The twinship experience in utero is commonly experienced as a conflict over resources, especially struggle for space, as one twin described:

> For me the physical sensations I relived in regression were very familiar and not frightening. My twin above me was a heavyweight; there was no room for me. Today I need a large house with high ceilings and glass. I also see how as a result of my intrauterine experiences I set up a victim relationship with men.

Ruch emphasized that the way we are conceived determines the way we are born. For example, in his personal experience, there was an imprint of the struggle to survive—either in or out—at conception, implantation, and birth. He recalls his experience of great difficulty implanting as the second fraternal twin. Physiologically the uterine wall thickens after implantation, which may make it a struggle for the second one to put down roots after the first. For Ruch it was one of "the most traumatic situations in my life—I am not going to make it, I have to die"—accompanied by strong physical feelings, wanting to scratch a hole into the wall with my hands."

Ruch suggests that many second twins die because of physiological difficulties with implantation. *In vitro* fertilization (IVF) research has shown that the greatest loss of IVF embryos, like naturally conceived ones, is in the uterus. Perhaps implantation rather than other aspects of the uterine environment is the problem, and particularly if more than one embryo is transplanted. However, I have observed that other twins have felt it was easier—the bed was ready with the covers turned down, so to speak.

The first half of Ruch's life in a soft, tender world began to change as he sensed his "kingdom" becoming "limited, even constricted . . . with a sense of "something" outside of him, far away, yet bumping him . . . sometimes at random, sometimes like a response, a shadow, like "two balloons slightly hitting one another." Initially, he felt playful and thought it would be fun to reach out to the shadow, but as he attempted to do this, he simply spun around in the fluid. His early impression at this stage was "something in between with no end and no beginning."

Later Ruch describes "a kind of a wall . . . many times I touched it, crawled up and down but I never found an opening." Wanting to reach out to feel and hug, even to rip open the wall, he found that their skins could never touch, there was "always a skin in between" preventing contact.

Disturbances of Ruch's prior oceanic bliss became more frequent, and were experienced as intense, even violent, interrupting his sleep. All the while he became progressively more confined, and being kicked and hit in his back made him feel "unprotected and vulnerable." With no possibility of escape, he felt forced to struggle, becoming increasingly angry and frustrated at the lack of space, which further restricted the expression of his discomfort.

I became more scared and threatened by my brother's appearance. We started to fight much more, especially if one of us tried to turn. I felt pushed towards the walls, and furiously started kicking and striking out as hard as I possibly could. Really I couldn't do anything to defend myself. The only way to express my discomfort was by kicking and moving my body. But soon I became exhausted and tired. I had no viable defenses to ward off the storm. I often gave up and fell back deep inside my body to find some peace and rest. . . . I became afraid of my brother's movements and sudden eruptions. He rendered me naked and unprotected, while I became tense and awaited another attack.

As a result the dilemma developed that these unborn twins could not relate to each other while both were fighting for space and struggling to survive. "My warm friend became an enemy and a threat. To survive I had to attack too, had to push him down." However, as Ruch was so powerless to resolve the situation, desensitization was his only option, becoming numb and less aware, as a cover for his inside hurt and frustration.

Through primaling these early experiences Ruch gained insights into his relationship with his twin. He had always felt a tremendous pressure to compete with his brother, at school and in sport as well as at home. He understood the reason for his competitiveness—it related back to a matter of survival. When this was relived and released, he felt free of this compulsion in his adult life.

Twins often corroborate prenatal experiences to their mothers. For example, "I was there when the egg split—That's how you got me." "You used to eat on top of me and Joey—didn't she Joey?" The issue of the firstborn twin, always foremost in the public's curiosity, can be set to rest by such remarks as: "Eric came first—I pushed him out, grabbed his leg and came after."

Physician George Engel, in describing his close bond with his identical twin, reported a "diffuseness of ego boundaries, never feeling sure who was who," and stated that he experienced a profound confusion between himself and his brother in dreams.

Understanding the dynamics of twin pregnancy through adults in regressive states led me to develop recommendations for parents of multiples. Prenatal bonding presents more of a challenge than with singletons, since the mother in particular must accept the idea of more than one baby and initially this often means bonding with the unit first. Next, differentiation is necessary to perceive each twin as an individual, without the ever-present temptation to place the twins at opposite poles when describing characteristics.

TWIN CONCEPTION

Conception events are fascinating when primaled by an identical twin, and especially in cases where both twins experience parallel events, unbeknown to the other, sometimes at the same time in different places. A therapist who specializes in twins told me about one of her clients who finally traced her feeling of being pushed around by other people back to being born as the first twin, but being kicked out rather than leading the way. A day or so later, her twin called to say that under hypnosis she had learned why she always felt she must struggle to get ahead and kick people around!

Two identical twins made separate but synchronous approaches for therapy with Graham. Both felt confused about their sexuality. One had been married, but had given up her son for adoption since she did not feel maternal enough to rear the child after her marriage broke up. The other twin was separated from her husband for reasons of sexual ambivalence. These twins began to primal similar issues, often at the same time, and sometimes even at different ends of the same room in group sessions. Individually, they both relived their conception as experiencing two sperm entering the one egg. Both separately experienced one sperm pushing the other one back out of the egg, then the fertilization and split into twins. The ever-so-brief presence of the second sperm, which was destined to produce a male child, was sufficient in their separate minds to explain their respective sexual confusion and/or bisexuality.

After making these connections, the more feminine of the pair returned to her husband and felt sure that she would keep any future child she might conceive. The other twin entered a very meaningful heterosexual relationship.

Another case involved an adventurous man who chose high-risk activities. When this man had a chance to take a hot-air balloon over Mt. Everest, he became terrified, feeling that this time he really could die. Intuitively feeling the need to primal his experience of splitting into twins, he flew 500 miles to work with Graham, within twenty-four hours of having this insight. His experience was captured on videotape, and a summary was published in *Aesthema*, the journal of the International Primal Association. He explained how he cloned his identical twin between the second and third cell divisions of the fertilized egg.

When I was on the floor at your place last time, I was trying to feel the reason for all this underlying anxiety that I have. . . . I've been coming to you on and off to have some courage to try and tackle it. . . . I started to feel what it was to be a twin. . . . I felt split in a way I've never felt before. . . . I felt split in my everyday living for sometimes I want to do this and part of me wants to do that. . . . At conception I feel that the conditions in the womb, perhaps the very reason for conception, was so painful that conditions in the womb weren't very good. My mother was sick, she smoked, and she drank alcohol. The only way to cope was to try to split off from myself so I could survive these alien conditions . . . long enough to get out in the world as early as I possibly could. Perhaps that is the reason I was premature. I didn't want to stay in there. The pain of life was so great that the only way to cope was to split into two people and that's what I did just to survive. In fact my twin didn't survive, he died at birth. . . . I believe from a crushed head but that's a whole other story. . . .

It's been the hardest moment in my life to re-create on the floor at the primal place. I know that my whole life has been directed from this time . . . that I live dangerously. I like to climb mountains, I like to kayak dangerously and fly balloons. I will probably do that for a long time to come. I don't know what the future holds for me in my everyday sort of living action. Perhaps if I can feel the full trauma of just coming into existence, that will change the direction of my life.

This man did get the courage to take his hot-air balloon to Mt. Everest, but the fuel ran out. Nevertheless, he went up 30,000 feet, higher than any other human being in a hot-air balloon, which was filmed in a documentary called "The Flight of the Wind Horse."

PRENATAL LOSS OF A TWIN

Rank wrote, more than seven decades ago, that many neuroses can be understood as an "embryonal continuance of the prematurely cut-off existence of a brother or sister." Often that sibling is part of a set of multiples. The earlier the period of gestation, the greater the likelihood of loss.

In the early literature on prenatal memories, before ultrasound technology confirmed the phenomenon of the "vanishing twin," the presence of a twin or double was thought to signify the placenta. Peerbolte insisted on this interpretation even when a client was sure an actual twin had been present.

The conflict over space and survival in the uterus may manifest itself in later life as issues of identity and creativity. A twin who sought psychotherapy from Arnold Buchheimer for blocked creativity came to understand that as a surviving monozygotic twin he could not feel whole unless he gave up, or blocked, part of himself. After therapy, he was able to take possession of his self and his space in the world without fearing that harm would be done to another, and his professional work blossomed.

Christopher Millar concluded from his regression experiences that he is a surviving twin. In his monograph *The Second Self*, he suggested that many famous writers and artists reveal their identity as a twin survivor through their work. Examples include Edgar Allan Poe's "The Oval Portrait," Dostoyevsky's novels, Lewis Carroll's *Through the Looking Glass*, Oscar Wilde's *The Picture of Dorian Gray*, Bob Dylan's song "Simple Twist of Fate," Paul McCartney's song "Yesterday," John Lennon's "#9 Dream," Leonardo da Vinci's *Mona Lisa*, Shakespeare's *Twelfth Night* and his "dark lady" of the sonnets, and Elvis Presley's song "I'm Left, You're Right, She's Gone."

Millar postulated that such artists' "creative drive results from experiencing loss of part of themselves. They are conscious of their immortality by being creative, an insurance that some part of them will exist after they are dead. Each creation is at once an attempt to regain their first creation, namely a copy of themselves, and an expression of their creative spirit which produced the copy in the first place."

I occasionally ask my workshop participants simply to draw a tree (with emotive music playing). When the group has finished, they are asked to look at the sketches with the tree representing the placenta and cord (a concept that was developed by Terence Dowling; see the guided visualization in Appendix 3). People draw fruit on the tree that exactly represents the number of children in the family, and the variety of shriveled roots, sticklike branches, sturdy trunks, full symmetry, and so on provide a symbolic smorgasbord. I recall one woman who announced that she had drawn *two* trees—one large and robust, and in the background a very small pine. I suggested the possible loss of a twin and recommended that she ask her mother if there was any bleeding or problems during the pregnancy.

Fascination with mirrors, facial asymmetry, and reflections, left-handedness, stuttering, and malformations have all been attributed more to twins than to singletons and may lead single adults to believe they once shared the uterus.

A psychiatrist once called me after he had learned, through guided regression in water, that he lost a twin at the blastocyst stage. He felt that his twin had been less able than himself to cope with their mother's ambivalence toward her pregnancy. He now understands why, as a physician, he avoids emergencies: they trigger his primal feeling of helplessness, just as he was unable to assist his twin who was calling for help before he passed on. We agreed that surviving twins have certain personality traits; for example, we never give up, to compensate for the twin that did. Interestingly, this man's wife was pregnant when he called (not such a coincidence at the time of his own prenatal quest). She was larger than usual for her stage of pregnancy and like most surviving twins, he was fervently hoping to have twins.

Loss of a twin at any time is tragedy; the powerful imprint of this experience in early pregnancy is sometimes more profound than the loss at birth or later. One reason may be the phenomenon of survivor guilt. Survivors of a twin pregnancy, unlike a plane crash or freeway accident, feel that something they did ("took all the nutrients or space") enabled them to live but caused their twin to die. Other dimensions of self-doubt include feeling the less deserving or the less wanted one (e.g. wrong gender). The following experience was described by a woman who lost a twin in the uterus. She was plagued by depression and insecurity in relationships, and was greatly improved after she realized that she was a surviving twin.

My conception was a struggle, a rape. The first three months I spent nurturing and desperately trying to save my twin. But in reality there was not enough room for two so I pushed my twin away, and she died. I spent the next six months hiding, not wanting to see what had happened. I didn't want to say goodbye to my twin. I had to be induced and needed forceps to drag me out.

My feeling of being a twin was of not having any space for me at all, of rigorously competing for that space and being at times enraged by this. There isn't anything there for me —no food, no oxygen, no space, and no special feeling because of my femaleness. As a fetus I am inert, but I try to eke out an existence in the top of the uterus sharing space with my brother who constantly thrashed about, kicking me in the head and body.

The crescendo of my fear is at its highest pitch at birth. I can hear them coming and I know that I am going to be born first and it should be my brother. His head is in the cervix and he is keen to go. By this time I am full of anesthestic gases and drugs, and my awareness becomes cloudy. I seem to be a spectator, in part, to what's happening to me. I feel myself being pushed and pulled and manipulated very roughly. I am dragged out of the uterus by my right arm and then hung upside down by my feet. My feet are being held very tightly and it's very painful. My head is then flexed back against my back and there are fingers in my mouth and a tube down my throat for what seems like ages. Then the worst thing of all happens—I am alone.

Graham Farrant believes that the vanishing twin syndrome is an emerging psychiatric condition. He describes one patient who, unaware of her twin history, always bought two items of clothing and another who bought a duplex house so the other side could be kept empty. Mothers of a surviving twin have reported various behavior such as the child talking to a make-believe companion, dreaming of a twin, or setting the dinner table for the nonexistent twin.

MaryEllen O'Hara, Ph.D., a psychotherapist and birth educator in San Diego, has no children yet but has suffered three miscarriages. All her life she experienced a feeling of "reaching toward someone" and had a recurrent dream that she was in a fog, with a piece of stretchy wall, "like plastic," between herself and the other person. She recalls trying to reach through it, wanting to grab and save the other. As a child, she often asked her mother if she had a brother; although she already had three brothers, she was always looking for a lost brother. Her mother suffered miscarriages six months before MaryEllen's conception and six months after her birth. During MaryEllen's gestation, her mother experienced bleeding and contractions between the fourth and fifth months. She had never discussed these episodes with MaryEllen who, much to her mother's astonishment, was able to describe exactly how her mother felt. Her mother remembers that MaryEllen reported her recurrent dream since the age of four and that as a child she often played with plastic, stretching it over her face and calling out. She was also fascinated with looking through glass, especially frosted glass or any silky, shimmery material.

In regression MaryEllen felt "weird sensations," and the right and left sides of her body felt different, lopsided, one side hot, the other cold. During one session she reexperienced the formation of her amniotic sac, "watching a balloon inflate and feeling it coming out of the middle of me, and spreading all around me, with each breath like a parachute or a sail. I was encased in it when done, like a larva in a cocoon." In both her recurrent dream and her regression she felt an "intense desire to unite with the other person." She sensed that he was a male, and her grief was profound when she experienced his demise. The experience of his leaving not only meant she had to be on her own, it was "earth-shaking, the deepest connection to who I was—the male part of me" was gone. She subsequently realized how difficult it had been all her life to accept her "masculine" qualities, such as assertiveness and success at her career. She felt that her excess weight was where she stored her grief.

MaryEllen's connection with her uterine experiences allowed her to acknowledge her feeling of deep loss and realize that she could not "find" her twin. Gradually the dreams went away, as did her avoidance of her masculine qualities. She concludes, "It was a turning point for me no longer to search but to live my own life fully and to have healthy, stable, male relationships without fear of abandonment."

The psychologist Carl Rogers once remarked that whenever he crossed a new frontier in his personal growth, it was as if a telegram went out to all his clients, because they would suddenly present similar experiences. I believe that the resonance factor plays a role in the kind of clients one attracts as well as "chance meetings" in life. At a workshop I took in Strasbourg last year, we were asked to go outside and pick up some item in nature with which we felt attuned and then tell a personified story around that object to our partners. I immediately found a broken stone and spoke of my loss of the other half. The French woman with whom I was paired became incredulous: she had always felt she was a surviving twin and had never told anyone. This was a powerfully healing interaction for her.

One of Graham's most extraordinary cases involved a woman, Sandra, who became paralyzed in her right side, as a way of representing her dead twin. She also wanted to make her mother feel guilty for much sexual abuse and an incestuous pregnancy that resulted when Sandra was a teenager. Sandra's paralysis came on after a lumbar puncture, but her physicians could never determine the cause. Subsequently in therapy with Graham, she relived her mother's attempt to abort her which had succeeded in the loss of her twin. (Her mother was unaware of a twin pregnancy; she assumed that Sandra was conceived right after the abortion and born early.) The needle in Sandra's spine several decades later triggered the paralysis, which was resolved when she connected with the memory of the knitting needle, used by her mother to abort Sandra's twin. This magnificent example of almost instantaneous "connection = cure" was filmed on videotape. Gradually Sandra's fingers began to move as the memories rose to her conscious mind. She regained full function of her left side as a result of accessing her primal reality.

In Sandra Landsman's *Found: A Place for Me,* a surviving fetus relives an abortion attempt of her twin which was verified by her mother. The scene was a room, in which she stood feeling unsafe. She experienced herself as one of the two pictures on the walls, watching in terror as the other disappeared.

As the second picture was about to be ripped off the wall, she tried to melt into the wallpaper . . . but someone was scraping the wallpaper off the walls. If she were to survive, then she would have to become part of the walls themselves. She froze as she disappeared into the walls. This became her perpetual state, the cold frozen immobility that she had lived with for so much of her life.

Leah LaGoy, a California psychotherapist and surviving twin, underwent chiropractic treatment for over a year. However, the pain in her sacrum immediately resolved when she relived the abortion of her twin. The instrument used by her mother had also struck her—on the sacrum. LaGoy's connection with this primal event had another positive benefit. By hanging on and surviving the attempted abortion of her, she felt that she "earned the right to be here."

There can be imprints from a lost twin right after conception, an experience of debilitation that one individual described as going through life thereafter "rowing with one arm." Laterality is an interesting phenomenon with surviving twins; in the few cases whom I have supported, the lost twin was on the left.

RESOLUTION OF HABITUAL MISCARRIAGE IN A SURVIVING TWIN

Sarah was referred to me because of her inability to achieve a term pregnancy, having experienced one ectopic pregnancy and (like her mother) three miscarriages by the age of thirty. Her medical history included every imaginable intervention from three dilatation and curettage procedures to karytoping the chromosomes of each partner. She was understandably very depressed and discouraged.

As I took a detailed history (and I ask *every* patient about her birth, gestation, and conception), I learned that the miscarriages always occurred between four and six weeks of gestation. Intuitively, I felt that something had happened to Sarah between the fourth and sixth week of her own gestation.

During the first session, she felt disconnected from her body apart from some nausea, and expressed much victim language. Ultimately, tears and anger poured forth over her myriad medical interventions. After a half-hour of inactivity in the second session Sarah went into deeper feelings, and responded that she felt as if she were "floating, dangling with a string through her middle." (Such metaphors may be obvious to us, but the patient may not realize that this is the umbilical cord.) Then came grimacing and grief reactions: "It is leaving to my left," and "I'm moving this way" (she slid slowly to the left). I asked her if it felt right to say "*I'm* leaving (wondering if perhaps her mother attempted to abort her). No, she replied, "I'm staying, I'm hanging in here. But I'm so afraid, and I don't want it to leave." I asked her if she was hanging on with her hands and feet, and she said, "I don't have hands and feet yet." Thus, I knew, that her embryological development was prior to six weeks.

In five more sessions she relived many prenatal events, including conception, which she described as a "splitting" (an identical twin). Her intrauterine existence was often expressed with much grimacing of the left side of her face and body, which tied in with her feeling that the twin was to her left. Over the four months that I saw this patient her demeanor improved markedly, and her painful periods (a symbolic cycle of life and death) and headaches abated.

When I asked Sarah at the first session what she thought her body was expressing through her symptoms, she had said, "My body doesn't let me walk away. . . . It's telling me 'I don't want any of these children.' " She now realized that conceiving embryos to replace her twin was the way that her body "didn't let her walk away" from that unknown primal drive that pushed to acknowledge and grieve for her twin. On that level she wanted her twin first and foremost, before "any of these children."

In her seventh and final session, she seemed to complete this stage of her bereavement for the lost twin, and I closed with a guided visualization of her uterus as a nest, together with affirmations of her ability to nurture a pregnancy to term. Two cycles later, she conceived for the fifth time and delivered a healthy baby at term. With no further problems, she later delivered two more children.

Surviving twins need to have their gut feelings taken seriously. It does not occur to singletons to fabricate such a situation. Survivors need to be acknowledged for who they are, to be "seen" as LaGoy puts it. Otherwise there is a general fear of annihilation especially in the case of an aborted twin, and a special fear that "mother will kill you all over again and no-one would know."

Since I understand the impact of twin loss in unknowing survivors, both personally and professionally, I encourage mothers to affirm the twinship of the survivor and acknowledge the death of the twin at anniversaries, discussions of pregnancy or birth, and other family events. Well-meaning health-care professionals, friends, and relatives should *never* tell the mother that she is lucky to have one living child, or that the other multiple's death was for the best, or other such pseudo-reassurance. A mother needs affirmation for her loss and grief, and support, as she goes through the enormously challenging paradox of bonding with one baby while at the same time mourning the loss of the other. This subject is explored in greater detail in the chapter, "Emotional Consequences of Twin Loss," in the second edition of my book *Having Twins*.

We have a much deeper appreciation today of the potential and the awareness of unborn and newborn babies. Next, we will address the challenges for expectant and new parents to create the most fulfilling and least frustrating environment they can during the primal period.

CHAPTER THIRTEEN

Prenatal Bonding: Children of the future

From the moment of conception until delivery nine months later, the human being is more susceptible to his environment than he will ever be in his life again.

—ASHLEY MONTAGU

Expectant parents need much education and support in today's increasingly medicalized world. The more they can identify with their unborn child's feelings, the more they can find the courage to "just say *no*" to unnecessary and inhumane practices concerning pregnancy and birth. However, they invariably need to clear their own personal issues first at a time when "vertical stressors" from the past intersect with "horizontal stressors" from the present. Pregnancy is thus an active dialog between the unborn baby, his mother and her psychosocial environment.

PERSONAL REALITIES

The exploration of individual reality in a regular childbirth class is limited. The issues, if not primal, are at least too personal and private to emerge in a large group meeting for short periods of time. Over the years I have offered both private counseling as well as intensive weekend "playshops" for couples. Often bonding with the unborn baby is challenged by a previous unnecessary Cesarean, fear of failure with the upcoming labor, guilt over an abortion, or grief over a recent death in the family. Sexual abuse, memories of which are often buried deep in the unconscious, can lead to major problems during pregnancy and labor. Sociologist Ann Evans found that if a woman had experienced sexual abuse by a caretaker prior to the age of eighteen, she was twice as likely to deliver before thirty-four weeks of gestation and two and a half times more likely to have a newborn with a medical problem. This occurred regardless of the number of previous babies, education, race, alcohol, cigarette abuse, or history of other physical abuse in childhood.

Time and again, the biggest gaps in people's conscious knowledge concern momentous life events, such as adoption; death of a twin, sibling, or parent; or serious childhood illness. Expecting a baby thus can enhance the healing of a family unit by allowing old issues to be explored and resolved, and even setting the family tree straight at times.

Recall of each parent's own pre- and perinatal memory helps them understand their formative experiences, as well as to value the consciousness of the child in the womb. A place to start is the questionnaire and genogram in Appendix 2, followed by the guided visualizations in Appendix 1.

Organic experiences are those felt through the body, and the musculoskeletal system is an easy place to begin. Stretching and strengthening exercises for couples to do together are described in the third edition of my book *Essential Exercises for the Childbearing Year.*

Partner stretches for the hamstrings provide the experience of pain and allow courage and tolerance to develop. "Playing with one's limits" to learn surrender is the best preparation for labor contractions. Sound may help to release the pelvic floor in birth. Keeping quiet usually means blocking the breath, which leads to tight throat muscles and further causes tension in the vagina, anus, and urethra. Moaning and groaning with the stretches helps both the mind and the body to yield and channel the intense energy of birth.

The pain of labor, I believe, is no more than resistance to the process of *opening up*, and this opening up happens on all levels: physical (cervix, vagina, and pelvis are stretched open), mental (the mother is taxed to her limits), emotional (primal feelings are stirred up), and spiritual (a conduit for a new being). But these ideas have to be experienced through the body, week after week and month after month. I have taught partner stretches for over a decade, and the feedback from mothers is that this valuable preparation enables them to stay with the process of labor.

Each parent can gain insights by writing a birth story, describing the upcoming labor and delivery as if it had already happened, preferably in the past or present tense. The biographical forms and birth stories make a special personal record for the couple. One woman read her story in an impassioned voice: "And as I entered their palace of technology, I vowed they would not separate the dancer from the dance." This was empowerment for her and for all those who listened.

Birth preparation modeled on our education system—filling up people with facts—has failed in most cases. Less than 10 percent of women give birth naturally, without drugs or instruments. Birth has been subtly redefined in recent years to fit the technological model; many now interpret "natural birth" to mean vaginal delivery! That is, as long as a Cesarean is not performed—despite the use of narcotics, epidural, forceps, or vacuum extraction—it is "natural birth." Such semantic confusion among professionals has set up a conspiracy that does women a serious disservice. Redefining the birth experience in this way is supposed to prevent women from suffering feelings of guilt or disappointment, but it eventually backfires. In their hearts women know the truth. Being "reassured" about unfulfilled transitions is a put-down that does not allow negative feelings to be expressed and affirmed. And then mothers feel even more guilty and upset over their angry or sad feelings if others judge their feelings as unjustified!

Educator John Holt, a pioneer of the home schooling movement in the United States, reminds us that:

We all have greater powers than we think. . . . Whatever we want to learn or learn to do, we probably can learn. . . . Our lives and our possibilities are not fixed by what happened to us when we were little, or by what experts say we can or cannot do.

CLEARING THE WAY:
PRENATAL COUNSELING

One expectant couple came to me for a private consultation because they were dissatisfied with their hospital childbirth classes. It was the second marriage for the husband, whose first child had been born at home, but the first marriage for the wife, Marcia. It is unusual that the man has had more experience of pregnancy and birth than the woman. Furthermore, Marcia's baby was breech and she was adamant that she was going to have a Cesarean. Marcia was not interested in being referred to an obstetrician who would try external version to put the baby in a head-first position or, if that failed, to deliver the baby vaginally. She insisted that she would never change her doctor. So I asked her what she would do if her doctor changed his protocol, and decided to deliver breech babies vaginally? By the look on Marcia's face, I saw that I had caught her out—she really wanted a Cesarean. Next I inquired: "Do you want to be prepared for a vaginal or a Cesarean birth?" Her answer was, "Both!"

I asked Marcia to relax comfortably in the bean-bag chair on the floor. She was apprehensive and reluctant to close her eyes. However, she cooperated well with a guided projection of the birth. She was able to give answers spontaneously to create a concrete setting—for example, the day of the week, the time of day, the room in which she experienced her first sign of labor, the clothes she was wearing, and so on. When it came to the pushing, I asked her, "What position are you in as you start to push out your baby? At this point she broke down into tears, crying that she could only remember the position that she knew the first wife was in when she gave birth.

I gently suggested that the baby had done her a great favor

by assuming a persistent breech position so that she could have an honorable Cesarean, and therefore would not be put in a position of competing with her predecessor. Both Marcia and her husband wept and embraced each other; this was their issue. Such a unique problem would never have been addressed in a class setting, and maybe not even in one of my groups. Whether Marcia went on to have a Cesarean or not, I never heard. However, if she did have a Cesarean, she consciously knows why. Her baby, however, had already begun his role of "fetal therapist."

Mehl and Peterson have described their phenomenological approach in their books (*Birthing Normally, Pregnancy as Healing, Mind and Matter*), and in Peterson's most recent *An Easier Childbirth*. Noting that attitudes, beliefs, expectations, and lifestyle interact with physical processes in the body, they observed the phenomena that appear throughout the process of a client's pregnancy. For instance, clusters of psychological attitudes may relate to a specific physical problem. If the individual can make connections, then resolution can occur before problems arise during labor. Positive images are programmed into long-term memory storage to recreate a different state when memories are aroused during actual birth. The woman must experience body sensation to become active participant in linking the processes. Peterson, Mehl, Klaus are among those who have used hypnosis and visualization to prevent premature labor, which Cheek described as a "preventable disease" because he, too, found that hypnosis can successfully stop contractions when the disturbance of the dynamic balance between mother and child can be understood. Since the prematurity rates for both singletons and twins have barely changed despite greatly increased medical intervention, prenatal psychology offers the most promise. Premature births occur in about 7 percent of the population, but make up nearly three-quarters of babies who die during the first month after birth.

PRENATAL ENRICHMENT

Rank suggested that sexual love reaches its climax in the mating of two beings, the attempt to partly reestablish the primal situation between mother and child, which "only finds its complete realization in a new embryo." The more we learn about the awareness and potential of the unborn baby, the more we can engage in sensitive communication with him. Recognition of the nature of the unborn infant contributes to his developing sense of identity and confirms that he is unique, with characteristics distinct from his parents and a twin, if present.

If the embryo feels his mother's moods and emotions, why should not the mother be equally affected by her unborn child's mental state? Fodor wrote that when the mother's blood turns cold (with fear) or hot (with rage), there will be endocrine disturbances in the mother (levels of which have since been measured). Fodor realized that if the mother hates the father, this is also communicated to the baby, who may grow up to share that hatred. He felt that the mother's fond expectations and reassuring thoughts may have a "very salutary influence on the psyche of the unborn child."

Gentle sexual behavior by the parents during pregnancy can produce pleasure reactions in the unborn, however any overtones of violence can be distressing. The baby often perceives the father as an attacker, the penis as invasive, and the weight as crushing. Kicking is the way a baby signals his protest or need for attention.

Touch is the first sense to develop and all other senses arise from it. A baby responds to touch by the seventh week, and by twelve weeks he can move his toes, feet, and legs. He responds to being stroked and caressed, and can learn to anticipate such interaction. Making contact in this way is also fun to do with a group of pregnant couples; they have the opportunity for feeling and deep connection with other unborn babies.

Babies move in rhythm to music and remember melodies from prenatal days, which can be soothing in the postpartum period when they are fussy. Studies have sought the kind of music that is optimally received by the unborn, and Mozart seems to be the winner. Odent instituted singing in his clinic outside Paris. Expectant and new parents gathered in the evening to sing and socialize. This served the dual purpose of helping mothers and their unborn babies feel happy, and providing an informal exchange of information about the childbearing experience.

Toward the end of my second pregnancy, I taught several training courses in prenatal and postpartum exercise. The tape I played for the postpartum aerobics was *Flashdance*, but one track in particularly imprinted on my son (so I learned after his birth). It was "Romeo," with the refrain "It's a boy, it's a boy, it's a boy." I had never consciously been aware of the words, until my son was about eleven months old and the tape was played at home, the first time he had heard it since his prenatal days. Although he could not yet walk, he stood holding on to a chair, and started to bounce up and down moving his hips and knees as if to dance when that song came on! I am convinced that he remembered my emotional state, as I greatly desired a boy. Unknown to me, I must have felt different when this track played, although consciously I don't really like that song and didn't even recall the words.

When the family talked to Carsten in my uterus, we would often introduce ourselves. We used touch as we spoke, and would play games that introduced words and concepts, usually singing, often in the bath or pool. For example, "Carsten's growing nicely inside. . . . Carsten's growing long and wide," or "This is up and this is down and this is round and round," placing hands appropriately. I believe that it is the personal interest, excitement, and interaction of the mother and other family members that provide the ideal prenatal enrichment, not technical equipment with prerecorded sounds. I have been deeply touched by a quaint phrase that my son began to use as soon as he could talk, "My good Mama, I want to *keep* you." It always sounds like his internalization of my prenatal projections!

I encourage visualization and contact with the baby on all

levels—physical, emotional, spiritual. Expectant parents can listen to the heartbeat of each other's babies, draw images of their unborn child, and share dreams, anxieties, and expectations. Prenatal enrichment evolves naturally when a mother has truly incorporated her baby, so that she blossoms from the center of her being.

UNRESOLVED ISSUES

It is helpful for each parent to verbalize his or her feelings to the baby. If a woman had attempted an abortion, or even made and canceled the appointment, it reassures the baby if she can stroke her belly and confess, asking for forgiveness and patience as she works through her negative feelings. Denial does not work; the baby knows because he is bathed in his mother's emotions at all times. Helen Watkins, a hypnotherapist in Montana, helps women who have decided on an abortion to experience less trauma. She guides a communication with the fetus so that the mother can grieve *before* the loss, rather than months or even years later. With emotional release, there is a reduction of guilt, which is important not only for the mother's psychological well-being but lessens the chance of another unwanted pregnancy. Sometimes hypnotic visualization even causes a spontaneous abortion; the mother asks the baby to leave and he does.

Unresolved feelings about abortions, spontaneous miscarriages, and stillbirths are common. Abortion may later give rise to a tumor or cyst in the ovaries, uterus, or breast, although few people make that connection. Guilt becomes sickness depending on the sensitivity of our conscience, it has been said. Miscarriages often express an unconscious purpose hidden beneath an excellent alibi; at other times the will to keep the child may triumph over the unconscious urge to destroy it.

Repressed feelings can be a major obstacle to normal birth and bonding, and my small-group format facilitates the sharing of these painful, often unacknowledged events. One woman got in touch with her suppressed guilt after losing her first pregnancy following a chorionic villus biopsy (a genetic test done in very early pregnancy). Expressing to the group that she felt like a "murderer" enabled her to grieve that loss and move on to bond with her present baby, which she had hitherto avoided.

Laing calculated that the majority of pregnancies are unplanned. It is therefore important to allow each parent to experience his and her own reality—resentment or fear about the pregnancy—rather than urge "positive thinking" or "being responsible." Then the shift may happen naturally, and perhaps without the development of complications.

Whenever I hear of complications in pregnancy and birth, I wonder what the woman was *feeling*, what was going on in her life. As rescuers leap in to fix the situation with drugs or instruments, I wish someone intuitive were present to explore the phenomenology—to look at the situation as symbolic, as expressing a human experience rather than a failure of the "incubator."

LABOR, BIRTH, AND POSTPARTUM

Pregnancy and birth are unique opportunities for the expansion of a woman's sense of self, a deepened trust in her inner wisdom, and a profound fulfillment from being connected to all life. Yet women are frequently dissatisfied, uncomfortable, or even afraid of their changes during pregnancy and birth. Too often, giving birth is seen as a problem to be solved rather than a unique reality to be experienced. The rhythms of labor are feminine to the core, yet the linear partogram that charts the progress of labor is a male construct. The demedicalization of birth should be followed by its demasculinzation, and this is not just a matter of putting women in men's jobs. Rather, we need attendants with a feminine principle, which Maine obstetrician Christiane Northrup explains as "values to live for" compared to masculine values "to die for."

Ceanne DeRohan, in *The Right Use of Will*, interpreted pain in childbirth as:

> just another expression of less than total attunement between the Spirit and the Will, and between the mother and the child. Total attunement never brings a painful or life-threatening situation to the birth experience.

Pain springs from resistance, repression, and blocking. All that needs to be done is to let go of resistance. Women need the kind of support from clinicians to surrender to childbirth that they would receive from therapists if reliving those same events in age regression.

In 1949, Fodor stated four basic principles that are still unheeded by most maternity units today:

1. Birth is traumatic in almost every instance.
2. The longer the labor, the more serious the physical complications, the greater the trauma of birth.
3. Intensity of the trauma of birth is proportionate to the shocks or injuries which the child suffers during labor or immediately following delivery.
4. The love and care which the child receives immediately after birth is a decisive factor in the persistence and intensity of the traumatic pressure.

Trauma in childbearing is often an echo of the trauma of the mother's birth. Imprinted on the organism is a complete record of reproductive activities. Childbearing becomes complicated whenever the similarity between giving birth and being born approaches the threshold of awareness. The dynamic tension of the memories stored in hidden recesses is apt to cause disturbance as soon as a parallel psychological state arises. Mothers know they are not likely to die, yet they may feel as if they were confronting death. If a woman identifies herself with the child in her womb, she may be as frightened as if she were about to relive her own birth. She loses the distinction between being a mother and being an unborn child; it is as if she were giving birth to herself. It was more than four decades ago when Fodor wrote:

> The life of many a child is lost because of this confusion in the mother's mind. The psychological education of pregnant mothers is sadly lacking. Of the relationship between their own birth and the birth of their child they know nothing. They do not even suspect that the child feels as if it were dying during a difficult labor, because they have forgotten their own birth experiences. Nature saw to it that the awful memory should be repressed. How, then, can they suspect that unconsciously they are dreading the recurrence of this terrifying event?

Chilton Pearce and Montagu stress positive functions of birth to prime the baby's internal organs for survival outside. Still, while the mother's afterpains are acknowledged and treated with pain relievers after delivery, no similar therapy exists for the child, nor is the need for it even recognized after a complicated birth.

A few years ago, the *Boston Globe* ran a feature story on birth, describing how a husband turned around a dysfunctional labor. While his wife was being readied for a Cesarean owing to "lack of progress," he leaned down to the unborn child and said, "Bozo, please come out!" And Bozo did! Obviously there had been a high degree of prenatal bonding between Bozo and his parents.

POSTNATAL BONDING

A mother's anger at a nurse or doctor at birth may be perceived wrongly as anger toward the child. In pregnancy the unborn child may blame himself for parents' unhappiness and decide that it is his responsibility to make his mother happy. It may be his idea to be born easily and not to cry. On the other hand, because of his disappointed expectations he may reject one or both parents and become detached. Babies have been born with stomach ulcers, and some refuse nourishment, especially nursing (although sometime they will nurse from another woman.) The message is: "I was so angry at my mother I didn't want anything from her."

Every child needs constant assurance of its own goodness and welcome, or self-rejection will follow. Pediatricians John Kennell and Marshall Klaus wrote their landmark work, *Parent-Infant Bonding*, in 1982, showing the importance of the period after birth for state-dependent learning and imprinting.

According to Klaus and Kennell, the mother's face conveys to the baby his worth and identity; newborns spend 80 percent of their time gazing at the mother. As Laing emphasized, the infant needs his mother's presence to fully live and move and "have his being." He cries when she leaves the room for, in a sense, his own being disappears, too. An infant whose separation experiences have created memories of imminent or actual depersonalization, even though repressed, will tend to be afraid at moments, such as when falling asleep, when there has to be a surrender of one's own awareness of self-hood as well as of other people. The family bed is one way to alleviate those fears and provide continuity of body contact for the child as he makes the transition from identification with the mother to personal relationships with others. Rocking, carrying, singing minimizes the change in existence from inner to outer worlds. Rhythm is the promise of a continuum; even as they grow older, children love to swing, ride a rocking horse and turn somersaults.

MOTHER POWER

Maternal love is the most powerful emotion I have ever experienced. One of the most joyful aspects of raising my children were the years spent sleeping beside a soft, little body, cuddling a small foot or hand. The sweet scent of baby breath is unforgettable. Instead of the baby crying from a crib down the hall, he wakes up in the family bed with a beatific smile and can snack at the milk bar whenever he chooses. Mothers who sleep with their babies are meeting the child's fundamental needs for food, security, touch, and love. The puppies in the pet store window are always huddled together enjoying body warmth and contact. Indeed, all mammals sleep with their young except affluent humans. Unfortunately, as Michel Odent notes, "for the last three centuries women have been told, first in the name of morality, and then in the name of science . . . that to sleep with their babies is a bad habit." He stresses also that the emotional-intuitive part of the brain reaches maturity before the age of two, making this primal period so critical.

It is time to break the conspiracy of silence about mothering. We women must speak about what is important for us and for our children—not what is okay, or even desirable, but what is essential. The time has come to let go of gimmicks like "quality time" or "natural childbirth with interventions" and speak the truth about bonding, birth, breastfeeding, and the family bed. Reich waged a lifelong campaign against the "emotional plague," which is what he called the social forces that repress natural, spontaneous, and of course sexual behavior. Historical change results from changes in child-rearing modes occurring through generational pressure. Each generation must thus speak the truth as it feels it in its heart.

What I call the *white bread philosophy* has undermined a century of common sense. Many of us know that whole-grain bread is better than white-fluff bread, but because it is harder to find and the hospitals don't usually serve it, we let ourselves fall into the trap of reassuring people that there is no real difference between white and brown bread. It is less of a hassle to acquiesce and take what is available. This is true for bread, and the analogy holds for a host of issues in women's health. Society says "It's okay to bottle feed" or "a Cesarean is no big deal; anesthesia is so good now and you'll be out of the hospital in three or four days," "it's easier to have your son circumcised now; it's cleaner and you won't have to worry about it later," or "kids in day care turn out just fine."

Under the well-intentioned guise of avoiding guilt, blame, and criticism, we have diluted the value of the childrearing experience. Every mother and baby is entitled to a deeply satisfying, transformative relationship—a magical rite of passage. By "equalizing" breast and bottle, and natural and Cesarean birth, the information, support, and real commitment to the way nature intended is greatly weakened. Women are told "whatever you want to do is fine." But it is not. We are creating the next generation, society's most precious resource for the future. It is time to point out that the "emperor is not wearing any clothes," that such "reassurance" rides on information that is wrong and harmful. Medical staff become co-conspirators, sometimes deliberately to assuage their own guilt feelings or unconsciously out of ignorance.

For poor, single, and working mothers these rights are not a choice; they are denied by circumstances. The problem is not, for example, breastfeeding, but lack of financial and social support to permit and encourage it.

While extensive maternity and paternity leave is necessary, more child-care subsidization is not the answer. Separating mothers and babies to create more woman power in the work force only adds to the social problems we have been discussing. As it is, more than 18 million children under the age of six spend more time in day care than with their parents. Mothers need to be supported in *mothering*.

Anxiety is the main source of violence, beginning as a gnawing sense of insecurity and rejection. The sadness of feeling alone, lacking a connection with others is established as an emotional predisposition. Even when things improve after birth, the child is likely to feel that "sadness seems more like the truth . . . I couldn't let go of it even when I was finally held by mother." Lack of bonding at birth creates fear and lack of trust, causing babies to grow into individuals who prefer the known environment of separation and even alienation. Research is accumulating that links the absence of positive bonding with addiction, co-dependency, criminality, self-destructive behavior, fear of intimacy, fear of parenthood, and the quest for security and self-esteem in the pursuit of wealth.

The Commission on Crime Control and Violence Prevention, created in 1979 by California state representative John Vasconcellos, recommended "alternative birth practices that include parental involvement, family intimacy and natural deliveries that discourage overuse of intensive care nurseries and labor-inducing drugs." Today's statistics reflect a trend in the opposite direction.

CHILDREN OF THE FUTURE

When a plant does not do well, we don't blame the plant. Instead we look to the garden and ask ourselves if it needed more sunlight or water, different nutrients or pruning. A child is like a plant. Children learn by imitation, and they "play back the tapes" relentlessly. They expertly comprehend subtle cues, unspoken gestures, and double meanings; what parents repress the child is sure to express. Chilton Pearce observed:

> We tell children how to be and instead they keep mirroring what we are. Children learn by example. If we are to raise happy children, we must bring to wholeness the models they are following. Be what you want your child to become.

We must recognize children for who they are so they will not need to camouflage their power and lose touch with their core self—the part that is intuitive, spontaneous, and authentic. Children are "equal in spirit but less experienced in form," said Shakti Gawain. We are the leaders because we know the territory a little better. But we must honor their autonomy and assume that they know who they are, what they want and need, and that they have valid feelings and opinions. Pearce continues:

> Unquestioned acceptance of the given . . . is the hallmark of the whole child. Anxiety over survival causes a screening of information through the questioning, "Am I safe?" The bonded child asks only, "Where am I?" and moves to interact accordingly.

Adults and children both respond to having their emotions respected and validated. In fact, it is because we were told as children to "not make a fuss" and "don't be a crybaby" that we disconnected from our feelings in the first place. Learning to feel emotion again, to respond freely, heals us to provide the same opportunities for our children. In fact, not to regain our insight and spontaneity leads us instead to blame, moralize, issue threats, punish, and react in other harmful ways when our kids press our buttons.

Parents in touch with their own emotions can be more tolerant and understanding of the healthy expression of negative feelings. Rather than label their baby as colicky, fussy, or difficult, parents need to facilitate the discharge of their infant's feelings, and not force them to be controlled and suppressed. It is more upsetting to a baby to be "shooshed" out of his or her emotions—perhaps a pacifier or bottle stuffed into the mouth, or even medication—than to be allowed his anger. Next time you are with a crying baby or small child, affirm his experience with such comments as, "Yes I know that hurts. I can see that you are feeling upset. It's okay to let us know what is happening." The child calms down and quiets much sooner with your validation of his reality than with your redefinition of it ("Be quiet" or "It's not that bad" or "You're a big boy now").

Sometimes I have observed my children misbehaving in ways that I believe they did not *learn* from me. But I recall behaving in exactly that way to my parents! If imprinting on the DNA of the pre-gamete cell is possible, then my eggs have passed on my childhood misdeeds to my offspring. In this way, the universe is giving back to me what I have put out; I don't need to wait for a future lifetime to suffer my sins.

We relive our childhoods in our children and we may recreate our childhood trauma by treating our children in the same way. This is why bringing prenatal and perinatal experiences to consciousness and making connections is so important. The optimist in me hopes that the next generation will bring about a kinder, gentler world.

CHAPTER FOURTEEN

Toward Social Transformation

Experiential work on prenatal and perinatal issues seems to lead to a new type of human being. Such a person has the capacity to appreciate and enjoy existence and shows deep spiritual feelings about the world. He or she has reverence for life, tolerance toward others, and understanding of interdependence in nature and society.

—STANISLAV GROF

Making pre- and perinatal connections can lead to fruitful social activism. Rank and Fodor saw all cultural accomplishments, such as art, philosophy, and religion, as a way to sublimate the desire to return to the womb. But as we have seen, the womb is far from a paradise, rather, it is often uncomfortable, tense, and even life-threatening. This aspect must also be taken into consideration when understanding human behavior and history.

Psychohistory is the history of the psyche seen in the context of the dynamics of large groups. The psychogenic theory of history involves the acting out by adults of group fantasies based on motivations initially produced by the evolution of childhood. The only new science to be developed in this century, psychohistory, offers untapped predictive and preventive potential. Lloyd deMause, editor of the *Journal of Psychohistory*, constantly monitors editorials, cartoons, and metaphors in the social and political arena and makes predictions based on his model of group fantasies, many of which are birth-related.

DRUGS, SUICIDE, AND
TEENAGE PREGNANCY

If we are to keep growing along with our children we must be able to regress to their pyschic age and work through the anxieties of that age, more successfully the second time around than in our own childhood. To be reborn means also to be reborn in our children.

A positive birth experience, bonding, and breastfeeding provide the best foundation for healthy child development. Likewise, there is accumulating evidence that prenatal and perinatal events influence social problems such as drugs and violence.

Bertil Jacobsen, M.D., at the Karolinska Institute in Sweden, found that addicts were more likely to have been born by mothers who were given narcotics and anesthetics, and that this was dose-related. Jacobsen believed that opiates, barbiturates, and other drugs given to women in labor made those infants more susceptible to drug addiction in later life. The first cluster of drug addicts in his study were born around 1945, which was when Swedish mothers in labor started to receive pain medication on a large scale.

Traumatic experiences at birth are imprinted, leading to a compulsive urge to repeat the trauma as an adult. The adoptee in New York who set the house on fire to burn his parents, or the rape and "wilding" of the Central Park jogger, are just a couple of examples that reveal the extent of rage among our nation's youth when primal affirmation is lacking.

Salk found that teenage suicide was related to birth trauma. Common factors were over one hour of respiratory distress at birth, mothers who were chronically sick during pregnancy, and mothers who had a lack of prenatal care before the twentieth week. Teenagers who had been in incubators suffer marked or severe emotional disturbance resulting from not only the premature birth but also invasive handling in the neonatal intensive care unit. Later, sleeping and attachment problems arise in adolescence when these early issues are recycled.

The overall suicide rate in the United States has tripled in the last thirty years. Every seventy-eight seconds an American teenager attempts suicide and sixteen succeed each day. Jacobsen found that methods of suicide and birth trauma were related. For example, people who asphyxiated themselves by drowning, hanging, or gas inhalation were four times more likely to have suffered oxygen deprivation at birth. Dublin and Benzel described the case of a depressed patient on an ocean liner who felt tempted to throw himself out of the porthole, but it never struck him that he could commit suicide by jumping overboard.

Over 1 million teenage pregnancies occur in the United States annually, costing over $18 billion and resulting in a loss of annual family income of more than $5 billion, according to a 1989 finding by the American College of Obstetricians and Gynecologists and the American Association of Family Practitioners. In 1990, over 300,000 babies were born with prenatal drug exposure (PDE). Every day in the United States, more than 1,500 teenagers start smoking. And unwanted births are increasing. In 1988, 40 percent of the births were unwanted, according to the National Center for Health Statistics.

The crisis is devastating. These unplanned, unwanted, and often drug-exposed babies will soon be raising their own children. Most teenage mothers today were born to teenage mothers, just as most physical and sexual abuse is committed by those who were abused. A vicious cycle keeps cycling.

NATIONAL AND GLOBAL REPERCUSSIONS OF PRIMAL PAIN

Lake described how a tight uterus constricted the unborn; likewise, tight boundaries put social pressures on adults. The primal process of shock, adaption, and exhaustion is experienced collectively as well as by individuals, thus it occurs in groups, institutions, and even nations. Lake's colleague, Reverend David Wasdell in London, warned that rigid restrictive boundaries in urban populations can cause regression to primitive levels of anxiety, similar to experiences of frustration that occurred in the months between conception and birth. Witchdoctors, shamans, and religious systems used to validate an individual's anxieties when they emerged under stress, and provide social rituals to permit abreaction and help integrate primal pain. Today, people are held together with pharmacological glue.

In his article, "Perinatal Roots of Wars, Totalitarianism and Revolutions," Grof pointed out that revolutions, although they usually represent some degree of historical progress, have to fail in their utopian efforts because "their external accomplishments are not accompanied by [the] inner psychological transformation that would neutralize the powerful destructive forces innate to human nature." The situation becomes progressively worse today because people are on the verge of global catastrophe.

The titanic aspect of overgrown technology, the sadomasochistic elements reflected in the escalating violence, sexual liberation, industrial pollution, political corruption, and satanic cults are all examples of how we seem to have exteriorized the elements of our deep unconscious and to have made them part of our everyday life. The symbols and metaphors become a threatening reality.

Fetal distress is traumatic and the fetus has no psychological defense mechanisms to handle massive anxiety and rage. As deMause put it, the fetus learns that his good feelings are often interrupted by painful feelings that he is helpless to avert, and his "once-peaceful womb slowly grows more crowded, less nurturant and more polluted, until it is finally liberated only by the battle which is the upheaval of birth itself." Such powerful imprints lead to repetition-compulsion in later life. Psychohistorians explain how leaders function as "garbage collectors" for the various repressed feelings of groups and nations. They provide channels for projected emotions that individuals are unable to keep bound by means of the usual internal defenses. Images of strangulation and oppression have occurred in speeches preceding war, such as Henry Kissinger's speeches on the Middle East crisis and John Kennedy's message to the So-viets at the time of the Cuban missile crisis. Grof made the point, especially about suicides and crime, that the transgression seems to provide for the person an "explanation and justification of the existing guilt feelings rather than causing them." For example, persons who want to drown or hang themselves feel suffocated or strangled *before* they commit the act.

The "imprinted" fetal drama, then, becomes "the matrix into which is poured all later childhood experiences," as the child works over the basic questions posed by his experiences in the womb. DeMause summarized some of the common scripts:

> Must all good feelings be interrupted by painful ones? Do I always have to battle for every pleasure? Will I have the support and room I need to grow? Can one ever really rely on another? Is entropy the law of my world, with every thing doomed to get more crowded and polluted? Must I spend my life endlessly killing enemies?

The drama of the suffering fetus, postulates deMause, is the deepest level of meaning of all rituals, religious or political, in all primitive, archaic, or historical groups, no matter how many elements are present from later life.

DeMause explored the basis of the fetal drama in history and culture, and outlined five elements: (1) Poisonous Placenta, (2) Suffering Fetus, (3) Growing Pollution, (4) Nurturant Umbilicus, and (5) The Cosmic Battle. The complete fetal drama with all five elements is seen even in prehistoric art from the cave at Lascaux, France.

The hero of this drama is always us—the innocent *suffering fetus* (second element), but as in the womb the traumatic ritual of suffering from the *poisonous placenta* (first element) and re-birth is reenacted, with every major life transition such as puberty, marriage, and death. Baptisms and circumcision repeat part of the drama. Historically, all major group events have required a repetition of the fetal drama, at the end of each year, at every spring planting, during harvest festivals and carnivals, before battles, and at coronations. In modern times, nations accomplish their cleansing by weekly Masses and periodic elections.

The central terror that underlies all group life, from primitive taboo to modern political paranoia, is that of *pollution* (third element): "All social order is upheld, no matter how irrational it may be, to prevent the imminent danger of pollution of group life by a transgressor," speculates deMause.

The single most common political symbol portrayed by nations about to go to war is someone grabbing a pole in the middle of his abdomen—ropes, or chains, or usually a flagpole—representing the *nurturant umbilicus* (fourth element). These images comprised one-third of all the political posters in deMause's files. The symbolism is obvious: a long flagpole (umbilicus) with a waving (amniotic water) flag (placenta) colored red (arterial blood), blue (venous blood), or green (tree of life).

The growing pollution of the group always ends in a *cosmic battle* (fifth element) between the heroic Suffering Fetus and the serpentine Poisonous Placenta. The central element of the battle is the sacrifice of the beast, whether it be the Russians, the Ayatollah, or Saddam Hussein.

DeMause's imagination can bring history to life by reviewing the facts from a primal perspective. John Kennedy had to be shot a year after the Cuban missile crisis failed to cleanse the national pollution and rage, and Ronald Reagan had to be shot a year after the Iranian hostage crisis failed to cleanse the nation. But Reagan didn't die and just one week later, the abortive assassination attempt was represented on the cover of *Time* with the single word *Abortion*. It is significant how the abortion debate fluctuates according to the chronology of the fetal drama. In the United States, where the topic of abortion consumes such an enormous amount of media coverage and legislative activity, the issues are clearly deeper than the sanctity of life. If saving babies were the issue, then the Pentagon could arrange bake sales to buy battleships and the taxpayers' money could improve the lot of mothers who are raising the next generation.

The nationalist group fantasy within which we enact the

fetal drama today worships a "national will" (measured by Gallup polls) as interpreted by elected leaders, inevitable growing pollution of this "national life blood," a collapse of the national will, and a sacrificial battle against a bestial enemy, often another nation, to cleanse the national blood stream and accomplish the rebirth of national vitality. Priests select segments of the population, usually youth and minorities (as in the composition of the fighting units in the Gulf War) to be sacrificed. The symbolic placenta in Teheran was protected (even pig grease was put on the flagpole), but the U.S. embassy was stormed, another sacrificial lamb.

While many will dismiss deMause's speculations, I intuitively agree with him that the world needs leaders who can understand that political struggles are akin to birth struggles and symbolic rebirths. We need politicians who can handle and raise to consciousness the dynamics of regression, and sustain reality-oriented decision making under conditions of increased stress. The adjustment of reality to the unconscious may be considered as the real principle in human development.

TOWARD A DEFINITION OF HEALTH

Health problems and military weapons are two of the major challenges of our times. In the United States, one baby in seventeen has a mental or physical defect at birth, according to the March of Dimes, despite the burgeoning medico-industrial complex and an increasing proportion of the gross national product spent on health care.

The human species is unique among animals in that humans can look back and forward: back to the pre- and perinatal phase and forward to its consequences. Yet, as Odent pointed out, it is a mistake to attempt "to solve short-term problems without taking into account the infinite complexity of the neurohormonal processes." Odent lamented the lack of:

practitioners who are . . . fully aware of modern neurophysiology and bioechemistry but [they] know that behavioral problems, some types of anxiety and some kinds of madness are in fact defence reactions which must be respected rather than masked. They also know that emotions are a way to modify brain chemistry and that emotional states are influenced more than anything by the social environment.

Odent attempted to define *health* rather than look at the various components of disease. He explored the effects of pre- and perinatal experiences on hormone production and neurological responses that persist in later life. His areas of concern included maternal anxiety on the unborn child, bottle versus breastfeeding, sleeping in the family bed compared with a crib, and the effects of lighting during the newborn period on the incidence of depression in later life.

Emotions affect the interaction among hormones and the nervous and immune systems; this sheds new light on autoimmune diseases. As I am writing this, a news bulletin announced that arthritis appears linked to the hypothalamus (a part of the primitive brain concerned with emotions) instead of just a problem with joints. Hay's *Heal Your Body* may yet turn out to be the pocket medical guide for the future!

Medical science has never been able to explain why, even in an epidemic, the majority of the population never comes down with the disease despite the same amount of exposure. Fear of disease (and the hysteria and panic around AIDS is a typical example) helps intensify the disease process, making people apprehensive and weakening in their immune systems.

British physican Edward Bach (originator of the Bach flower remedies) wrote of the state of harmony that mind and body must achieve to "make it difficult or impossible for disease to attack us, for it is certain that the personality without conflict is immune from disease." He recommended that:

if we can only set aside a short time every day, quite alone and in as quiet a place as possible, free from interruption, and merely sit or lie quietly, either keeping the mind a blank or calmly thinking of one's working life, it would be found after a time that we get great help at such moments, and, as it were, flashes of knowledge and guidance are given to us. We find that the questions of the difficult problems of life are unmistakably answered, and we become able to choose with confidence the right course.

People need to free themselves from their self-created entanglements, to simplify their lives. Elisabeth Kübler-Ross advised:

Learn to get in touch with silence within your self and know that everything in this life has a purpose. There are no mistakes, no coincidences; all events are blessings given to us to learn from.

We must take responsibility for our own health rather than waiting until we get sick. As surgeon and writer Bernie Siegel discovered, the exceptional cancer patient is one who doesn't just decide "not to die" but makes a conscious effort *to live*.

Continued research into the development and interaction of the sensory equipment of newborns, their reactions and behavior, pre- and perinatal learning, and birth memories of adults as recalled in psychotherapy, is of great value. However, society, like maternity units, will be slow to recognize and honor the real importance of the primal period, until the power of pre- and perinatal imprinting is *personally* experienced or witnessed.

A major stumbling-block is the general human tendency to react with repression to any recognition of the "fetal drama." As a feminist, I appreciate Rank's insight that women have been put down both socially and intellectually on account of the original connection with birth trauma. He suggested that the female genitals (and all that emanates from them) tend to be denied and disregarded because of primal repression. We see this in health care, too.

Feminist Sonia Johnson, author of *Going Out of Our Minds*, reminded us that:

Since what is possible is whatever we can feel as fully as if it already exists, what we most have to fear is failure of the heart. . . . When we seize power in our inner world, the outer world will have to change.

Since all systems are internal systems, all genuine revolutions are internal revolutions, revolutions first and foremost of feelings, which translate inevitably into revolutions of values, of beliefs and of behavior. All bona fide revolutions are of necessity revolutions of the spirit.

DEVELOPMENT OF INTUITION

The psychic Edgar Cayce was once asked how intuition could be trained. He replied, "How would you train electricity—save as to how it may be governed!" Cayce indicated that intuition was a function of the soul.

Intuition, a highly significant part of traditional cultures, has been declining in the West with the increase in industrialization. Rituals and traditions that affirmed individual knowing have technological substitutes today that attempt to provide a fake "shared reality"; for example, watching television instead of conversing or seeing a birth film with all the props of labor but none of the essence of birth. The ever-expanding media, the common culture, and big business promote this fictitious reality, which also results in personal as well as political disempowerment, together with emotional and moral paralysis. Freedom to make choices in line with one's own sense of values becomes difficult, because values grow so perverted as a result of the all-pervasive influence from the message makers.

Feedback from others and the world outside lets us know how things are working out. But this must be meshed with internal feedback from feelings, and a sense of being alive and empowered. When we consistently suppress and mistrust our intuitive knowingness, looking instead for authority, validation, and approval by others, we give our personal power away.

This leads to feelings of helplessness, emptiness, a sense of being a victim, and eventually anger and rage—and if these feelings are suppressed, to depression and deadness.

We must not underestimate the power of thought, from the placebo effect to the evil eye. Planets affect each other even though millions of miles apart. When medical and scientific journals publish studies showing that patients prayed for by their cardiologists did better than those who did not have the benefit of prayer, and that seeds in a saline solution (normally lethal) will grow with long-distance visualization, we can see that change is around the corner.

A union is forming between the two models of the universe. The mechanical, reductionistic view and the holistic perspective are merging to create transformation. In my own education, and that of most Westerners, the pursuit of knowledge was paramount. Thoughts were valued more than feelings, logic rather than intuition, content more than process. American anthropologist Margaret Mead once said she was brought up to believe that the only thing in life worth doing was to add to the sum of accurate information. Pearce warned that acquisition of content is an obsession with adults who have no matrix. He advised:

> in a universe in which everything must move and flow in order to exist, only ability to interact with that flow is of value . . . information is of value only as it enhances the ability to interact.

Mystic Meher Baba taught that "in the absence of the illuminating wisdom of the heart and the clear intuition of spirit, intellectual perspective gives only relative truth—bearing the ineradicable stamp of certainty."

Much of automated modern life is a recreation of fetal existence; endless connections to tubes, wires, and equipment in all aspects of our lives, *but this time with control.* If we didn't like negative umbilical effect, well now we can select a soap opera on the TV and feed that in. But the more we use and depend on machines, the more we become like them.

Buying into the "shared reality" spares us from having to deal with our own personal reality or that of another individual. Reality is personal, as Einstein pointed out, always beginning and ending with individual experience. A person can imagine anything but can only *feel* what has been experienced.

Although intuition threatens some individuals' reality structures, this inner knowing is just as necessary in today's complex, contaminated, and chaotic world as in former times. How else is a child to know when to refuse a stranger, if she can't feel that "something is not right"? How can we predict if someone is a threat to us, physically or sexually? How can we make authentic choices in relationships if we are not in touch with our deep needs? How can we be true to ourselves if we are not aware of our true selves?

The American Society of Dowsers offers an annual conference and training school, and a quarterly journal, all of which provide information and insights about subtle influences on human behavior that range from electromagnetic fields and toxins to ancient monuments and energy lines in the earth's crust. Dowsers typically help others in a fruitful search— whether it is for ground water, food allergies, or missing items. The practice of this skill helps refine intuition, phrase a question in its essence, and contact higher dimensions of human awareness. Asking "May . . . Can I? . . . Should I?" develops an appreciation of the interrelationships in the universe. Parents, physicians, teachers, and government leaders would do well to ask themselves the same questions.

EVOLUTION OF PERSONAL ETHICS

It is a law of the universe that what we create within us is always mirrored outside of us. When you truly give up trying to get something outside yourself, you often end up having what you always wanted! We must see that the world outside reflects what is inside of us—poverty, violence, pain. Concentration camps, for example, are manifestations of certain aspects of the unconscious, and as deMause and Stephen Levine have both said, in their own ways, "Recognize the Hitler inside of yourself and then you can begin to understand." Then we can better *be* peace than try to *make* peace.

I quote the following passage from Edward Bach in its entirety to preserve the magnificent prose of his convictions. He was not referring to the healing power of regression, but I believe that experiences which enhance personal reality can help us to live life as Bach recommended:

> Next we must develop individuality and free ourselves from all worldly influences, so that obeying only the dictates of our own Soul and unmoved by circumstances or other people we become our own masters, setting our bark over the rough seas of life without ever quitting the helm of rectitude, or at any time leaving the steering of our vessel to the hands of another. We must gain our freedom absolutely and completely, so that all we do, our every action—nay even our every thought—derives its origin in ourselves, thus enabling us to live and give freely of our own accord, and of our own accord alone.
>
> Our greatest difficulty in this direction may lie with those nearest to us in this age when the fear of convention and false standards of duty are so appallingly developed. But we must increase our courage, which with so many of us is sufficient to face the apparently big things of life, but which yet fails at the more intimate trials. We must be able with impersonality to determine right and wrong and to act fearlessly in the presence of a relative or friend.

RELIGION AND SPIRITUALITY

Humans are unique on earth in that they can contemplate the cessation of their existence. Grof observed that the only way individuals can deal with existential anxiety is through transcendence. Primal journeys lead not only back to the self but may carry one to transpersonal dimensions and cosmic awareness. In her book, *Living in the Light*, Shakti Gawain describes her passage "through darkness," in language rich with birth metaphors:

> But the darkest hour IS truly just before the dawn. When we finally give up the struggle to find fulfillment "out there," we have nowhere to go but within. It is at this moment of total surrender that the light begins to dawn. We expect to hit bottom, but instead we fall through a trapdoor into a bright new world. We've rediscovered the world of our spirit.

David Mintner, a facilitator at Graham's clinic, explained how the primal experience heightened his sense of self-worth.

> Many, many times I started with "It's hopeless. I'm just no good" and after a painful journey through my thoughts and emotions, ended up with something like, "It's amazing, I'm part of every thing. There's nothing to be afraid of." Contact with that profound place has gradually transformed my life. But it shocks me when I look back, how resistant I have been. Until recently I have stubbornly refused to understand the true nature of my base. It's almost as though the transformation has taken place despite "me" (what I normally think of as "me").
>
> Formerly, I was severely limited by fear of life, fear of death, self-loathing. . . . I cried and raged and shook, and slowly began to identify with more attractive parts of me, with what I felt positive about rather than with what I feared.

Regression often helps individuals avoid investing their "inner knowing" in someone else—gurus, teachers, bureaucracies. People on the inner quest can move away with ease from the partisan position of institutionalized religion. Jung believed that the main function of formalized religion was to protect people against direct experience of God. To enable people to unfold the potencies of the soul aspect is to put them in harmony with the forces and energies hidden in nature.

Meher Baba clarified the role of mysticism:

> Spiritual experience has a grip on deeper truths that are inaccessible to intellect. . . . The fact that spiritual experience involves more than intellect alone can grasp is often emphasized by calling it a mystical experience. . . . Mysticism is frequently regarded as opposed to intellectuality—obscure, confused, impractical, unconnected with reality—but in fact true mysticism is none of these. There is nothing irrational in true mysticism when it is, as it should be, a vision of reality. It is a form of perception that is absolutely unclouded, so practical that it can be lived in every moment of life, and so deeply connected with experience that, in a sense, it is the final understanding of all.

RELATIONSHIPS AND SURVIVAL

Lake felt that to become mature we must counter the dangers of overdetached isolation and overdependent union. We suffer not only from separation anxiety but also from commitment anxiety; we are liable to be immobilized because we dare not let people move away from us or move too close, threatening the integrity of our invisible boundaries.

As victims, people enlist rescuers to save them. Rescuers do not know how to take care of themselves, so they focus on healing others, unconsciously trying to fulfill their own needs in an indirect way. A rescuer believes that others are weak or powerless and need his help. You can't be a rescuer, said Gawain, unless you believe in and have a victim inside.

When individuals are rescued, they sense this unconsciously; it serves to undermine their power instead of helping them find their strength. More importantly, as rescuers we are not taking care of ourselves, which will move energy and transform the situation. Taking care of ourselves means trusting and following intuition by listening to all our feelings, including the hurt feelings of the child inside, and responding with appropriate action. Gawain emphasized that we must put our inner needs first and trust that as we do this, everyone else's needs will get taken care of and everything that needs to be done will get handled. Saying "no" may support a person in finding his or her own power instead of giving in to their powerlessness. Gawain explained:

> When I communicate truthfully and directly, and say everything I really want to say, it doesn't seem to matter too much how the other person responds. They may not do exactly what I want, but I feel so clear and empowered from taking care of myself that it's easier to let go of the result. If I keep being honest and vulnerable with my feelings to my lover, family, and friends, I won't end up with hidden needs or resentment.

Healthy relationships are based not on neediness but on the passion and excitement of sharing the journey to becoming a whole person. If we let relationships reveal themselves to us, they will take us into deeper levels of ourselves, and a stronger trust of the universe, and a deeper intimacy with others (to the extent to which we are prepared to be vulnerable). People who divorce feel they have failed whereas, as Gawain pointed out, actually the marriage has been a success. It helped the couple to grow to the point where they no longer need its old form.

VISION OF THE FUTURE

U.S. Senator Claiborne Pell once remarked that "primal attitudes toward life and death set the ethical environment and the possibilities for peace." *Psychic numbing* refers to the decreasing response (desensitization) and powerlessness that accompany increasingly stressful dilemmas—for example the teenage pregnancy epidemic, escalating social violence, or the proliferation of nuclear weapons.

Likewise, Chilton Pearce observed: "What we have done is develop an intellect that is devoid of intelligence. . . . That is why we have 500,000 brilliant scientists spending their time developing armaments." What happened to reverence for life?

As Fodor pointed out, we cannot be certain what happens to us when we die, but we may safely say that at one point we have been in definite contact with the infinite, at the time of conception, within the womb. According to Fodor, "the measure of organismically remembered perfection is the very drive behind our restless search for happiness and our ceaseless struggle for betterment." Our longing for the paradise lost, the symbiotic link with mother, or the vanished twin may spring from a buried connection to the divine.

People have to own their own pain and stop dumping it on others. As Hephzibah Menuhin said, "freedom is choosing your burden." When one's rage about emotional starvation by parents is expressed, a place can be found for appreciation and compassion to flower. "Take your life in your own hands, and what happens?," observes Erica Jong, "a terrible thing: no one to blame."

When we can each take back our own personal responsibility, the consciousness of the group can be raised. If fewer individuals act out their fetal drama, then there will be less imput for group fantasies and projections, which in today's nuclear world could quickly turn into a ghastly reality.

The heart is the most fully developed of all the organs at birth. But for most of us, we are split off and out of touch with this core of our being. Regression experiences, through the variety of approaches described in this book, may free a person to direct his or her consciousness toward the deeper dimensions of the self—the aspects that demand greater integrity of thought and feeling. Within the rediscovered matrix of life and love, it becomes safe to have a heart again.

Afterword

A Quantum Leap to Global Consciousness

—BY GRAHAM G. FARRANT, M.D.

When I accepted Elizabeth Noble's challenge in 1985 to venture forth from the safe confines of my own clinic to lecture in the United States, I genuinely never believed it possible that within five years I would "retire" from that place. Significantly, I gave my Australian clients and my clinic staff nine month's notice (the length of a pregnancy) of my intention to leave the center I had pioneered so many years ago. I had felt my way through all the personal feelings inevitably entwined in such separations, so that now I feel an exquisite sense of freedom, expansiveness, wholeness, and warm enthusiasm for the future.

Over the years my staff and I have observed an increasing number of clients who initially come into therapy for either physical or mental problems and who end up being specifically concerned about spiritual issues in their lives. Maybe at this time in the world, more and more people, at an earlier and earlier age, are becoming aware that we all live in a global village, and that we need to be concerned about the decline in moral integrity—right action toward all life. It is no longer sufficient to have personal integrity (being true to oneself, one's feelings) and complete health; we also need to be infused with a planetary consciousness.

I have come to rely totally on my inner knowing rather than

intellectual knowledge with regard to people's problems. I have come to believe firmly that the only true source of genuine resilient healing is unconditional love. Most people want to be listened to, to be genuinely heard on a deep, meaningful level of compassionate understanding and helped to find their own essence.

Unconditional love is a difficult ideal. It is hard for people to give what they didn't get, and when the unconditional love and nurturing of the uterine environment is lacking, it is difficult for the offspring to provide it for the next generation. Reconciling unconditional love with setting limits and saying no is always a challenge. Bernie Siegel, the famous Yale surgeon and writer about exceptional cancer patients, said that the ability to say no is essential for the immune system. It is important for me to set limits for unreasonably needy or disturbed people, to empower them in their own process rather than rescue them. However, I like to think that it is one of my advantages to be so open and sensitive at a cellular level, even if one of the complications of such openness is an inevitable vulnerability.

Let me give a personal example of the difference between the way I used to respond to a patient with classic depressive symptom expressed in the often-heard jargon, "What's the purpose of life? What's the point in living? What's it all about anyway?" In the past, I would have conceptualized these remarks as epitomizing, at a birth level, a depressed, perhaps long labor superimposed on an unplanned, unwanted pregnancy, with even a preconception sad egg syndrome. Now I would answer their question directly, by saying something like, "The purpose of your life is the same as it is for all of us: Namely, to get back in touch with your own divinity." Often I remember their eyes light up in the midst of their haze of depression. As one woman exclaimed so clearly and maybe on behalf of all other similarly afflicted souls: "That feels right. Why hasn't someone said it as clearly as that to me before now? What work do I have to do to get back to that truth?"

Instead of being locked in to the establishment view of psychiatric depression, including even my personal cellular consciousness construct, there is this other way of viewing depression: that it is nothing more or less than an awareness of separateness from God.

A New England obstetrician surveyed 20,000 fellow OB-GYNs on the following question: "What in your obstetric practice stresses you the most and how do you deal with the stress? He presented the results at the 1986 Conference of the International Federation of Obstetrician-Gynecologists in Melbourne. Of the 2,000 replies he received, by far the most common answers were fear of litigation and interviewing pregnant women. The doctors dealt with their stress by taking longer holidays and engaging in more recreational activity. Not one of the respondents volunteered, or even mentioned, any counseling or psychotherapy, let alone deep regressive psychotherapy. I followed this obstetrician's presentation with one of my videos, showing obstetricians and midwives who had reexperienced their births, dramatically altering their practices as a result.

A classic example concerns one obstetrician who routinely put forceps on every first-time mother until he remembered and realized the emotional experience that he himself had been delivered by forceps. Unwittingly, he was obliging every first-time mother to feel the same experience as an unconscious way of avoiding the experience of his quite considerable forceps pain at birth.

Professor Carl Wood, of Australia's Monash University and Queen Victoria Medical Center, did a decade of research to measure minute amounts of fetal oxygenation after birth, not realizing that he was motivated by personal experience of having had no oxygen during and shortly after his birth. And as a direct result of this connection, he told his residents and registrars to stop routinely aspirating every newborn baby.

Another obstetrician initially came to therapy because of constant fatigue and escalating disinterest in his career, mounting marital problems, and workaholism. He had become renown in his state for his knowledge of breech presentation and his apparant uncanny judgment in advising women as to the safety of a vaginal delivery. Very quickly in his own regression work he reexperienced having being born breech with one arm extended tightly over his head, with resultant temporary paralysis of his arm. He enjoyed a significant set of connections that enabled him to alter his practice significantly. His workaholism was directly due to, and an expression of, the effort he needed to get born. Because of his prolonged labor, he avoided ever feeling stuck again in his life, by setting his practice up so that he is always leaving one place to go to another. For example, he was always getting out of one consulting room into another or going from one country office to the others. This, of course, is time-consuming and physically exhausting. Once he had had the courage to feel that original physical discomfort of his breech birth, he was able to close three of the four country practices, reducing his fatigue and workload so he could be at home more with his family.

Over the years I have had the opportunity, even the privilege, of having many nurses and midwives in my workshops. I am prepared to say that in 100 percent of cases, when they regress to reexperience their own births, they always come out of the experience with the exclamation: "My god, that's the very point in a birth where I blank out . . . where I lose attention . . . where I interfere with the natural flow of labor." The commonest experience for midwives is to begin to feel agitated, restless, and impatient when labor goes on past a certain time. Then they unconsciously stop being supportive and caring, and become increasingly intrusive, even invasive. Again, this is all because of their own unresolved birth pain and diminished oxygen, with its consequent adult equivalent of "I don't know what's happening . . . I feel confused . . . something's got to be done." When these nurses and midwives have the courage to reexperience their own fetal distress, their behavior in the delivery room dramatically alters. When they are no longer triggered by what is happening to the present birthing mother and child, they don't inflict the same consequent trauma on the child being born.

As a step in addressing the problem of emotionally un-supportive medical personnel, my pediatric colleague John Spensely invited his final-year medical students to experience personal deep regression as part of their medical training. This was on a voluntary basis and only a small percentage of the class ever came. However, those who did always spontaneously regressed to an earlier repressed childhood experience. Many were also able to reexperience some aspect of a traumatic birth, such as a lost twin, Cesarean section, tight cord around the neck, and fetal distress. The majority of these students be-came general practitioners, and many of them subsequently re-ferred patients to resolve birth trauma before these patients conceived a child. Quite a few of the physicians actually elected to come back to further their own personal growth, with great benefit.

In my opinion, psychiatry has been plagued for decades with the unfortunate stigma of mental illness and derogatory diagnoses—labels that haunt people for years and drive them into family secrecy, social isolation, and self-fulfilling prophe-cies. The uniqueness of regressive work is that it reaches back to preverbal events. Counseling which is limited by language cannot help clients come to terms with the complex emotional trauma of birth or pregnancy, or feelings that may have existed in one or both parents at the time of conception. Deep regres-sion is a natural process. It works readily and easily for over 80 percent of people who embark on it. It is not a long, drawn-out process, and some results can be quite dramatic. Life-changing insights and connections can be forthcoming from even a one-day workshop.

If children were only allowed and encouraged in school and college to discuss their feelings in a constructive, supportive, and creative atmosphere, approaching therapists for help to resolve issues like birth trauma would become as natural and stigma free as it is to go to a physical therapist for a sports injury. One of the inevitable generational conflicts is the pos-sibility that some mothers will choose to feel guilty about what happened to the children they birthed, and some offspring will choose to protect them from that by not broaching the topic for fear of causing distress. If society is to change, and humanity is to avoid the steady decline in moral integrity and increase in violence and other social problems, then sooner or later one generation has to stand up and be counted. As Harry Truman had posted on his desk, "The buck stops here."

The expectant mother has the challenge and responsibility, but also the opportunity, of maximizing the potential health of her unborn child, by dealing with all her unconscious and unresolved psychobiological issues as far back as preconception. If you are six months pregnant and reading this, you will be in a position to compare the personality, character, and behavior of the child you will give birth to with that of any subsequent child you may bear in the future. I hope that between the birth of this child and your next child, you will take the opportunity to explore unresolved issues to maximize the potential of future children.

These days it seems easier for young women to talk to their mothers about their own birth and what it was like for their mothers to be pregnant with them, so at least they can start with an intellectual appreciation of any trauma that may have occurred during their uterine life or at the time of their birth. Because it involves a more open and frank discussion of the mother's sexuality, it is sometimes more difficult to talk about conception. But approached sensitively, it's possible to obtain a lot of useful information. And for those people whose mothers have died, or for adoptees or offspring of donor insemination and other types of reproductive technology, there is always primal therapy, cellular consciousness workshops, and other forms of facilitated regression.

An awe-inspiring video project, *Touch the Future* by Michael Mendizza, will bring together the combined wisdom of fifty of the world's authorities on human potential. When I spoke to Mendizza his quiet passion for his project was emphasized by his use of the word *urgent*. There is indeed an urgency in bringing the information in this book to the general public. The incidence of violence, drug addiction, and crime is escalating at such an exponential rate that, unless something profound happens to slow down this demise of humanity, American life will deteriorate into social decay.

The challenging issues that Mendizza's video project addresses are similar to this book. What is the role of affection in the healing process. What is love? What is the heart-mind connection? Is there a nonverbal channel of communication between parent and child that transcends thought and emotion? How can parents become more sensitive to bonding processes? What have we discovered about children who failed to bond or become attached? What are the damaging effects of being born unwanted? Can we prevent further damage from occurring? Can affection repair what has already taken place? What new therapy modalities have emerged to deal with the pre- and perinatal trauma? Where do we go from here?

There is no doubt that the practical, commonsense, down-to-earth advice, suggestions, and information poignantly expressed in this book will lead most readers to seek their own culturally determined pathway to appropriate and meaningful help. By resolving their lifelong patterns established in the very earliest moments of life, the endless generational repetition of pointless pain can once and for all be stopped. Raising children who experienced minimal pre- and perinatal pain will bring pleasure and wisdom to the parents and a joyful family, and a more harmonious society will be created.

Guided Visualizations for Pre- and Perinatal Experiences

The following two visualizations may help you access early memories. I developed the first one, which covers the journey from egg and sperm through to birth and meeting the parents. The second one specifically concerns the placenta and was written by British psychotherapist Terence Dowling. You can have someone read the sequences to you or record them on a cassette tape. My creation, *Inside Experiences: A Guided Visualization*, is available in several languages on audiocassette with specially composed music (see Resources for information).

GUIDED VISUALIZATION: CONCEPTION TO BIRTH

This guided recall is designed to arouse prenatal and perinatal memories. It is not necessary to read the headings—they are merely for convenience. You may want to have paper, crayons, and a tape recorder nearby to record your personal impressions afterward.

Most people are born vaginally. However, guided cues for breech and Cesarean births are at the end of the chapter, and can be inserted in place of vaginal birth. Then continue with the rest of the visualization from "Entering the World."

Note: Suggestions for women who are pregnant are in parentheses. You might wonder if this visualization is advisable to do during pregnancy. Sometimes images and feelings emerge that are upsetting, but in my experience of guiding pregnant women with this visualization for more than a decade, the rewarding resolutions that usually follow more than compensate for the unpleasantness of dealing with "old business." Often this work clears the way for a better birth experience, which is one of the main reasons to use this visualization during pregnancy. Always reassure your baby, if unhappy feelings arise, by explaining that these are *your* feelings and experiences, and are in no way caused by your baby.

Visualization is a powerful, but also self-regulatory process. People will not go against their own scripts—authenticity prevails. For example, a person may feel beyond all doubt that he or she was born breech, even during guided imagery for a head-first birth.

If something comes up that is too difficult or painful, you can step back and watch what is happening as would an observer, or simply just set it aside for now. Falling asleep is a protective mechanism, and not uncommon in individuals whose mother was actually "put to sleep" with anesthesia during the labor. Important feelings will come back, perhaps in a dream or when you play the tape again. The advantage of the audiotape is that you can play it whenever *you* feel safe and ready to go to deeper levels. When the apple is ripe, it falls from the tree.

Relaxation

Choose a position of comfort, preferably on your back (unless you are pregnant), with your arms and legs uncrossed. Feel free to move in any way at any time, as your body responds to the imagery described. Trust any hunches, intuition, and flashes of insight. Stay with any feelings that come up, and go with any desire to express yourself with sound or movement.

Begin by closing your eyes and listening to your breathing become slower and deeper, feeling yourself completely supported by the floor. Raise your eyebrows to stretch out any tension. Close your eyes and feel them heavy in their sockets. Allow your jaw to be slack, with cheeks soft, lips together, and teeth apart. In your mind's eye see your face at peace, expressionless, as you are breathing, a little deeper, all the way down to your feet and toes.

Bring to your mind a peaceful favorite place—the beach or a meadow, for example. Imagine that you are lying down in that scene, warm, supported, and relaxed, enjoying the particular sounds—perhaps the birds, the waves, the special smell of the grass or the sea—feeling the sun warm on your skin. You are trusting the earth to support every part of your body, so that no muscle work is necessary.

Become aware of which nostril is open right now—they alternate through the day. With each inhalation, allow your waist to loosen, so your diaphragm is free to rise and fall, and feel how it does this automatically. (Allow your uterus to soften so that the muscle walls can yield to your baby's movements, giving him/her lots of space to move and stretch.) As you become more relaxed with each breath, continue to breathe out any tension all the way down to your feet and your toes. Let any tension fall away down the strands of your hair. Let the relaxation spread down over your forehead, so that any lines on your face can drift further and further apart, releasing all the way down to your mouth, jaw, and throat.

Let your throat yield and be open—open to the air, to feeling (making room for your baby in your womb). Let any tension fade away with your outward breath. Make room inside for your organs, creating more space for your heart, lungs, internal organs; becoming softer and looser, relaxing right down to the base of your spine, and the muscles in the floor of your pelvis; just yielding to the rhythm of your breathing, in and out, in and out.

Now begin to imagine what your body looks like from the inside: blood vessels, nerve networks, joints, muscles. Notice how you always keep breathing. Your unconscious mind is taking care of all your internal bodily functions—your lungs, liver, pancreas, kidneys, heart—all functioning beneath your awareness. (Most miraculous of all is the growth of your baby, day by day and hour by hour, growing with its own wisdom and the wisdom of your body, without books, classes, or handouts.)

As you know, we all began as an egg and sperm that united. Our bodies formed and grew in our mother's uterus. Now you are going on the same journey again, down into your unconscious mind and getting in touch with some of your deepest feelings around the nature of those events.

Allow yourself to sink down into an even deeper state of relaxation during your next seven breaths. Count these seven breaths as you inhale through one nostril and exhale through the other and then repeat this with the opposite combination, taking all the time you need, breathing at your own rhythm, having an image as well as a sensation of the air entering in one side and leaving the other.

With each breath out, allow yourself to sink deeper and deeper into relaxation, letting go of tension, fatigue, and unwanted thoughts with each exhalation. Releasing, softening, yielding, surrendering. Sinking deeper, deeper down, way back in time. Stay with the rhythm of your breathing, in and out, in and out, relaxing your mind, relaxing your body—deep down, feeling very, very relaxed.

Back to the Uterus

I am going to count now from ten back to zero, and when I get down to zero, become open to the experience of floating inside of your mother: ten-nine-eight-seven-six-five-four-three-two-one-zero.

Allow your skin to feel the warmth and buoyancy of the amniotic fluid that surrounds and supports you. You are totally immersed, warm and secure. Let an image come to mind of your size, of your head and of your body, at this moment. How much space is around you? How does it feel to turn and stretch? Feel the walls of the uterus around you and the quality of contact as you touch them. Let your tongue taste the amniotic fluid. Allow your ears to hear the sounds inside the uterus: your mother's heartbeat, her intestinal rumblings, her voice. What sounds do you hear from outside—your father's voice, a sibling's voice? Maybe your mother played a musical instrument or used some equipment? Let your ears hear it again.

Allow yourself to experience the variety of emotions your mother feels while she is carrying you. What is her primary emotion that comes to you? Every memory is stored, and we carry the imprints of these early experiences throughout the rest of our lives. Today, let yourself access these feelings and sensations.

Now allow yourself to experience again *your* primary emotion as you grow inside your mother. How do you feel about your gender? And how does your mother feel about it? And your father? What about the timing of this pregnancy, for your mother, for your father?

What is your feeling about the purpose of your life? Why you are here? Do you have a sense of your destiny at this point in time? Did you choose your mother? For what reason? Did you choose your father? Why? Whatever images and emotions come up, allow yourself to stay with them and explore the bodily sensations. Feel the containment of the walls of the uterus all around you and how you respond to it. Feel your umbilical area. What is coming in to you as well as the oxygen and nutrients? Live again your primal reality.

Let your eyes see the shadows, light, darkness, any colors. Are you alone in the uterus? Is there any kind of disturbance in this oceanic, buoyant bliss? And if so, what size are you when it happens?

As you know, you began with the union of an egg and sperm, and I'm going to count from ten back down to zero so you can go deep down into your unconscious mind and get in touch with your earliest feelings as egg and sperm. Ten-nine-eight-seven-six-deep down-five-four-three-way back-two-one-zero.

Allow yourself to have an image of your parents during your conception. See their faces, their body positions; feel their emotions. Are they aware that they are creating a new life? Stay with any images, tastes, and smells that come along. What time of year is it, what time of day? How is the external environment, the weather?

Be aware if this mother is the same mother who later raised you. And if this father is the same father who raised you. Allow yourself to explore your parents' emotions. Whose emotions come to you first—mother's or father's?

Let yourself go right back and deep down into which every memory is easier to access—the feeling of being a sperm or an egg. Whatever comes up. Stay with the feelings and the sensations, trusting the process.

Sperm Memories

Every sperm starts as a tiny cell, maturing in the testes. Feel back to the time when you were suspended in solution, pushed along tail first by a special nurse cell, into the transport duct to a storage place at the top of your father's testicles. What is your journey like as you leave your father's body, jet-propelled in just a few seconds through the twelve inches of his genitals? Feel yourself becoming active in the semen, and feel the lashing movements of your tail, which is almost all of you. Become aware of this male energy, the drumming vibrations of the hundred million or more sperm around you. How does it feel to swim up the mucus channels in the vagina, a 10 km journey relative to your size? Experience the forest of cilia beating downstream as you swim against them. One thousand tail strokes drives you just one centimeter. Have a sensation of the speed at which you are traveling—or any rests or detours you take. Where are you in relation to all the other sperm? Are you aware of the uterus contracting around you?

Do you turn right or left as you enter the uterus and swim toward the opening of the tube? Do you already know what you are going to find? Is there a sense of magnetic resonance and attraction? And how does the egg appear to you, the largest cell in the human body, many many times bigger than you, a tiny sperm? What kind of choice do you experience around this egg you are approaching? How does it feel as you burrow into the layers of cells surrounding the egg? Let your sensations and emotions emerge.

Egg Memories

If you find it easier to access your egg memory, let yourself go back to the very beginning, the ripening follicle in the ovary. But which ovary? Right or left? Feel your outer layers of membranes and cells, and the experience of dividing, halving the number of chromosomes. And the feeling as you burst out of the follicle, then being guided and wafted along by the fringelike projections of the Fallopian tubes, down into the narrow tube. Which tube are you floating down—on your mother's right or left side? Do you already sense all the sperm waiting to meet you? Are there any other eggs going before or after you? How do you feel when all the sperm surround you? Who does the choosing? Let yourself experience the quality of the union.

Fertilization

As you know, at the moment of fertilization the head of the sperm explodes and releases the DNA, the genetic material in its nucleus into the egg. Feel the coming together of the two nuclei, staying with any feelings in your head or elsewhere in your body. Does your mother know she is pregnant at this moment? What is her response?

Cell Division

Twelve hours after the twenty-three chromosomes of both egg and sperm unite, the first cell division takes place. You pause, . . . your cells divide a second time. Is anything happening with your other half, the polar body? Cell division continues every twelve to fifteen hours. So you become two cells, four cells, eight cells, sixteen cells, thirty-two cells, and so on.

Allow yourself to witness the creation of your body, your cells expanding and dividing. Experience the pause between the cell division, as you start the long journey of three to four days down the narrow six-inch tube, slowly turning from the combined force of the remaining sperm beating their tails. Which way do you turn? Feel the downward flow of fluid and the waves of contractions of the tubes around you helping you along.

As you drift down the tube, do you have a sense of where you are going? Of what this life is all about? Of why you are here? Why now? Why these parents?

Now you have grown to over 100 cells, and are passing through the narrowest part of the tube just before the entrance to the uterus.

Implantation

Experience again your dropping out of the tube into the large, deep, dark void. How is your landing? Feel the outer transparent sheath around you shedding away, allowing you to develop further as you implant directly in your mother's uterus. Does your mother know she is pregnant with you as you connect for the first time with her body? What is her reaction? And your father's reaction—how did your mother tell him? Hear the words she said. In what area do you choose to set down roots? Feel the fingerlike projections connecting you with your mother's uterus. You are nourished by a yolk sac as well as the lining of your mother's uterus.

Your cells know exactly how to differentiate—their inner wisdom guides them to form liver cells, kidney cells, nerve cells, muscle cells, bone cells. Allow yourself to experience this creation as your body grows cell by cell. Let any feelings about your existence, your purpose, your awareness of the universe come into focus.

Feel your body forming the umbilical cord and the blood vessels connecting you with the placenta. As your cord leaves your body, which way do the blood vessels twist? Experience the pulsing in and out and the feelings you have about this rhythm.

Three weeks after fertilization you are an embryo, with your first nerve cells forming. At eight weeks you are now a fetus, one and a half inches long, with all your organs in place and your fingers and toes moving. By eleven weeks, your liver and spleen are working and your yolk sac disintegrates now that your placenta is fully functioning. Hear the sound of the blood as it perfuses your placenta. How do you feel about this genetically identical companion? How does it feel to your touch?

Your eyes develop by fifteen weeks, but remain closed until the seventh month. By the third to fourth month your hands can grasp and your feet can kick. By the fourth to fifth month you can hear the sounds of your mother's circulation, her intestines, her voice. You are floating inside a bubble surrounded by the membranes. Feel the pulsing of your umbilical cord as it slips between your fingers. Become aware of the area between your shoulder blades, which so often makes contact with the walls of the womb around you. How is the quality of that touch? How does your skin feel?

Are your mother's emotions changing as you grow? Whatever you sense, allow yourself to *feel* it. Hear the words that she uses when she talks to you, and about you. All these feelings and experiences are embedded in your mind. Let yourself recall them. If any painful feelings arise, remember that deep down there was a level of biological cooperation between you and your mother, permitting your existence.

Onset of Labor

As your body grows larger and larger, the walls around you become tighter. How do you respond to your space now? And what is it like to move and turn? Allow your hands and feet to move in any way you want right now. Feel where your head is in relation to your mother's pelvis. What is your response as the contractions become more frequent and active, the walls of the uterus around you pressing and releasing, squeezing and pressing and releasing, stronger and stronger as the day of labor approaches, getting near the time of your birth into the world. How do you feel about this timing? And how is the timing for your mother? Did you initiate labor? What season of the year is it? What time of day is it? Keep trusting whatever comes up. And as the contractions become closer, harder, and longer, allow yourself to feel the pressure on your body, from your feet all the way to your head, as you were squeezed down by the muscles of the uterus—those strong muscles that pull open her cervix. The contractions fade away like waves reaching the shore. Another contraction builds, presses, squeezes, and you feel yourself moving deeper down, deeper down. You feel the ring of the cervix opening around your head. And the contraction fades away; time to rest.

Feel your heart pumping faster, your adrenals pouring out their hormones. How is your oxygen supply right now? And how is your mother responding to active labor? Who is with her?

Vaginal Birth

Trust and honor your inner world of knowing as you live again your birth experience. Another contraction builds, squeezing and pressing. Feel the pressure on your head as the cervix is pulled open, open, all the way open, and your head slides through into the soft, stretchy folds of your mother's vagina. And the contraction fades away.

Feel when the membranes break and the amniotic fluid is released. Experience again the rhythmic contraction and expansion, contraction and expansion. Feel the direction in which your body wants to move. How is your energy?

And another contraction is coming, building, squeezing, pressing, molding your skull bones, shaping your head as it turns through the contours of your mother's pelvis, as you sink deeper down, deeper down. What position is your mother in? Become aware of any taste in your mouth, any sensations in your head or feet.

Another contraction squeezes and presses you down deeper. You feel her pelvic bones against your head. To which side does your head want to turn as you rotate through your mother's pelvis? Stay with any sensations anywhere in your body.

Another contraction builds, pressing and squeezing, down deeper, deeper; squeezing, turning, and pressing, down down; feel another ring of tissue, stretching, stretching; feel the floor of muscle you're passing through. Stay with the sensations and emotions as another contraction builds, presses, and squeezes, bringing your head down under the pubic bone, stretching, stretching your mother's vagina over the back of your head. And the contraction fades away.

Where is your cord right now? Are you doing this alone? What are the sensations on your head?

Another contraction is building, squeezing, and pressing as you dive deeper down. Feel your mother's vagina stretching, stretching as the tissues slide over the back of your head. Feel the air, feel the ring of tissue slipping over your forehead, nose, and chin. Your head is out, in the world!

And another contraction building, strongly squeezing, pressing against feet and body. Feel which way your head and shoulders turn, feel which shoulder is coming out first. Experience the rotation in your body as your shoulders are delivered one by one, and the rest of your body slides out.

Entering the World

Who catches you? How do those hands feel? What do your eyes see first as you leave your mother's body? How is the temperature, effect of gravity and air on your body. Allow your mouth to sense the very first thing that went into it. What is your mother's response now you are just born?

Allow yourself to feel deeply the many experiences of being completely outside your mother. What is placed around your body? What do you smell and taste? Is your father present? What is his response? What sort of room are you in? Who are the people present? What are the first words you hear as you enter the world? What other sounds? With the first breath, part of your old circulation shuts down and all the little sacs in your lungs fill with air. Feel that first breath.

Stay with any sensations and emotions that come up, especially around your umbilical area. What is your response when your cord is cut? And after you are separated from your placenta, where do you go?

Parental Contact

Allow yourself to remember the first time you were held by your mother and looked into her eyes. See her face, hair, clothes, but most of all see the expression on her face. And your father. Feel the first time he held you and looked into your eyes. What is his emotion? How do you experience your father's touch, how he looks at you, the sound of his voice?

If you had to do it all over again, would you choose the same uterus in which to grow? Whatever issues emerged for you, remember that you, a new life, sprang forth from deep levels of co-creation. Let yourself imagine an ideal welcome into this world. How would you like to greet a newborn?

Become aware of any assumptions you have made about yourself and your new territory . . . focus on any judgments and personal laws that resulted. If any of these images and memories today brought up feelings of loss, sadness, or anger, know that as we mature we can often look back at this formative time and see that they were valuable lessons. You may have an image of the person with whom you associate some negative emotions, and just for today you, or perhaps just a part of you may want to forgive that individual. Just let any resentment go, release old painful feelings, if you can—perhaps even if just for today.

Closure

Gradually focus your mind on your breathing and my voice, coming back to the present, being aware of the room and the sounds around you. See if you can wiggle just your left big toe while keeping the others still. And now move your right big toe. Gently wiggle all your toes, now. Starting to move your ankles, gradually bring the movement up to your knees and your hips, then gently rock your pelvis. Stretch one arm all the way over your head. Stretch your fingers long and bring that stretch all the way down through your wrist, elbow, shoulder, waist, and leg so that you are longer and longer on that side. And now stretch the other arm, fingers long, bringing the stretch all the way down to your feet and toes on that side.

Now stretch your right arm and your left leg, then your left arm and right leg. Drag your jaw down and stretch it from side to side; yawn if you want to. If any part of your body feels tense, stretch it just like a cat, slowly and luxuriously. If you are on your back, bend one knee and drop it over your straight leg to roll onto your side. Open your eyes when you are ready and take your time to sit up.

Cesarean Section

Allow yourself to recall whether you experienced any labor contractions prior to your Cesarean delivery. Is this a scheduled or an emergency operation? What is the mood of those around you? How is your mother feeling?

If you feel or know that your Cesarean birth was scheduled, allow yourself to experience the time before. Do you have any sense of an imminent event? How do you respond to the opening of the uterus? If yours was an emergency Cesarean, experience again the period right before. How is your oxygen supply? Your heart rate? How are you fitting in her pelvis? Where is your cord? Allow yourself to know the reason for this Cesarean.

Feel the sensations as the drugs and anesthetics are administered. Is it general anesthesia, and your mother is completely out? Does it bring a taste to your mouth? Perhaps your mother has an anesthetic just in her spine, and you can still hear her voice? How is the sense of timing for you as the doctors begin to cut? What are your sensations as the membranes are cut? Is the cord around your neck or any other part of your body? How is your breathing right now?

What part of your body is presenting in your mother's pelvis? How are you lifted up? Is the doctor and the assistant male or female? How do the hands feel? On what part of your body are they? Which arm is brought out first?

Feel what is happening with your mouth, your chest, your breathing. What is the position of your body as you leave your mother? Where are you taken now? What feelings do you have about the Cesarean? What emotional connection do you feel to the people around you?

Breech Delivery

Allow yourself to feel if you chose to present as a breech. Is there some reason why you are lying like this? What position are your legs in, and which part is engaged in your mother's pelvis? How is the length of your cord?

Feel the contractions building and pressing you deeper into the pelvis. Where is the pressure building on your body?

Experience your passage through your mother's pelvis. Do you turn to your left or right? Do your arms drop down first? Which arm comes down first? Be aware of how your neck and shoulders feel. Is there anything in your mouth? Feel your ears, your head, your chest, your breathing.

GUIDED VISUALIZATION USING THE PLACENTAL SYMBOL OF THE TREE

1. You walk toward a wall, and in the wall there is a door. Look carefully at the wall and the door, and remember what they are like.
2. Now you open the door. How difficult is it to do so?
3. You go through the door and you enter a garden. What sort of garden is it? Look carefully all around it. What is the weather like?
4. In the middle of the garden there is a tree. What sort of tree is it? How big, how strong, how many branches, how many leaves? Are there any fruits or flowers? What is the trunk like? What is the earth like around the tree?
5. Now you climb up into the branches of the tree. You can see the whole garden. Below your feet, there is a little hole. It goes right down the middle of the trunk into the roots. You go down this hole head first. What does it feel like? You go down into the roots of the tree.
6. Now you are in the roots. What are the roots like? How do you feel down here in this place? What is the earth like? Can you hear, see, smell, or touch anything?
7. Now you come up out of the hole. You come out into the light and the fresh air. What does it feel like?
8. Now you climb down out of the tree and stand in the garden

and look at it. Suddenly, something happens to the tree.
What happens to the tree?

Commentary

A healthy tree standing in a cemetery or on top of a grave
has often been given by a person whose mother suffered a
bereavement during pregnancy. An unhealthy tree in a grave-
yard has been given by those who suffered an attempted abortion
or threatened miscarriage. An unhealthy tree may be correlated
to fetal distress and trauma. Root size often indicates something
about fetal nourishment. The quality of the soil is also indicative
of general maternal emotional health during the pregnancy. If
the mother has smoked, for example, it is most often expressed
here by a bad taste and small tight roots.

What happens suddenly to the tree in the fantasy generally
reveals aspects about the loss of the placenta. Feelings of loss,
constriction, panic, defeat, anger, or liberation can accompany
the event which befalls the tree. When nothing is remembered,
and nothing is projected to the end of the tree, it is often a
sign of fetal narcosis or loss of consciousness at birth caused by
other factors.

Questionnaire and Genogram for Expectant Parents

Name _____ Age _____

Number of Pregnancies _____ Number of Births _____

Own Birth History _____

_____

_____

Breastfed? _____ How Long? _____

Own Conception History _____

_____

Birth and Gender Order (e.g., 2 sons, myself, 1 daughter) __

_____

Same-Sex Parent's Age at Your Birth _____

Same-Sex Parent's Age When Last Child Born _____

Same-Sex Parent's Health Problems _____

_____

Give a History of This Pregnancy _____

_____

Describe This Conception _____

_____

Previous Pregnancies and Conceptions _____

_____

Life Crises _____

_____

Please Attach a One-Page Autobiography.

FAMILY GENOGRAM

Construct a family genogram to explore more closely your family patterns, anniversaries, illnesses, and other aspects of family time. A genogram is a family tree with all the missing pieces—miscarriages, abortions, separations, affairs, divorces, accidents, and diseases.

The Symbols

⟨A⟩ = adoption

○ = female   □ = male   _____ = marriage

_ _ _ _ _ _ = affair   ◁ = miscarraige/abortion

/ = separation   // = divorce   ✕ = death

△ = vanishing twin   ⩕ = vanishing triplet

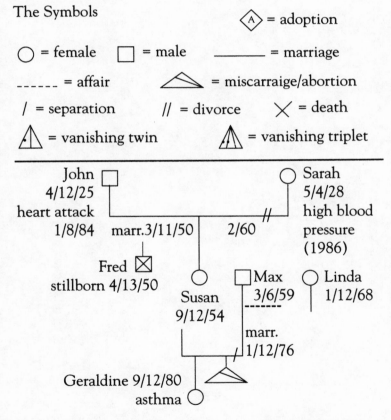

Example: Susan had her first child, a girl, at the same age as her mother (twenty-six), and separated at the same age as when her mother divorced (thirty-two).

Glossary

Autonomic Nervous System A part of the nervous system that is concerned with the control of involuntary bodily functions.

Blastula An early stage in the development of the ovum.

Blastocyte A stage in the development of the embryo, which follows the morula.

Embryo Stage of development between second and eight weeks.

Endometrium The inner lining of the uterus.

Fetus Stage of development from the third month until birth.

Gamete A reproductive cell, sperm or egg.

Morula A solid mass of cells resembling a mulberry, resulting from segmentation of the ovum.

Neocortex The convoluted layer of the cerebral hemispheres of the brain, the newest development evolutionarily.

Neurotransmitter Chemical messenger substance in the body that links nerve networks.

Peptide A compound containing amino acids.

Zona Pellucida Inner thick, solid, membraneous layer of the ovum.

Zygote The cell produced by the union of two gametes—the fertilized egg.

Resources
Finding a Facilitator

Here I have listed individuals and organizations who guide people in regressive experiences. Facilitators usually are therapists—trained in psychiatry, psychology, or social work—however simple humanity can be as important as professional training. Some of the best facilitators have learned by practical experience rather than theoretical instruction. Having undergone their own healing process, they can knowingly support others. For example, there are degreed professionals who offer regressive therapies, but who have not accessed their own birth or prenatal life. Carefully question therapists about their own personal experience and avoid them if they don't practice what they preach. Trust your intuition and choose a guide with whom you feel safe, and then the process will unfold organically for you.

INDIVIDUALS

Aquagenesis Workshops. P. O. Box 7134, Jupiter, Florida 33468-7134; (407) 575-0547. Prenatal regressive therapy developed by Sandra Landsman, Ph. D., psychologist and transactional analyst. T-shirts, prenatal affirmation symbols and charts.

Jeanne Avery. 88 Friar Tuck Lane, Ancramdale, New York 12503. Astrologer who assists clients in regression, through birth to past lives, to bring aspects in a horoscope into an experiential domain. Author of *Astrology and Your Past Lives* and *Astrology and Your Health*.

Jeannine Parvati Baker. P. O. Box 398 Monroe, Utah 84754; (801) 527-3738. Author, founder of Hygieia College, and co-director of the Six Directions Foundation. Consultation, workshops, books, tapes, videos on optimal family and planetary health via catalog, private appointments, congresses, symposia: "Healing the earth by healing birth."

Paul Brenner, M.D. 1330 Camino Del Mar, Del Mar, California 92014; (619) 792-8721. Former obstetrician offering preconception, prenatal, and postnatal counseling for individuals and couples. Life-events counseling for menopause, surgery, illness, bereavement and so on.

Cabine de Maternage. Anne-Marie Saurel, Villa Doube France, 6 Av. Des Acacias, 06800 Cagnes-Sur-Mer, France. Based on research by Tomatis (see Centre Tomatis) Anne-Marie Saurel developed a "Cabine de Maternage," in which the mother-child bond could be reconstructed using therapeutic techniques of audio-psycho-phonology.

David B. Chamberlain, Ph.D. 909 Hayes Avenue, San Diego, California 92103; (619) 296-7535. Psychologist specializing in hypnotherapy, hypnotic recall of birth and womb memories, emotional clearing of memories in preparation for childbirth.

David Cheek, M.D. 1140 Bel Air Drive, Santa Barbara, California 93105; (805) 569-7161. OB/GYN psychosomatic medicine, offering individual therapy and workshops in hypnosis, specializing in pre- and perinatal issues, especially with the infertile couple. Use of hypnoptic techniques for discovery and reframing of emotional issues.

John Diamond, M.D. Cantillation Research Foundation. Drawer 37, Valley Cottage, New York 10989; (914) 561-

8245. Australian psychiatrist and author of *The Body Doesn't Lie* and *The Remothering Experience*. Training courses and workshops in Cantillation: "Highest Form of Life Energy."

Terence Dowling, Ph.D. Kurt-Schumacherstrasse 95A, 6500 Mainz-Gonsenheim, Germany. (06131) 465825. Therapy designed to awaken or increase the client's awareness and understanding of their pre- and perinatal experiences and the role they can play in daily life. Hypnosis and analysis of muscular reactions in psychodrama are also used.

William Emerson, Ph.D. 4940 Bodega Avenue, Petaluma, California 94952; (707) 763-7024. Psychotherapist offering training programs for resolving prenatal, birth and neonatal trauma in infants and children. Maximizes human potential through reconstructive therapy and spiritual work with infants, children, and adults.

Jane English, Ph.D. P. O. Box 7, Mt. Shasta, California 96067; (916) 926-2751. Consulting and support for Cesarean-born people and their families, and for therapists working with Cesarean-born people.

Michael Gabriel, P. O. Box 8030, San Jose, California 95155-8030; (408) 993-9536. Hypnotherapist and counselor specializing in pre-birth experiences.

Kelduyn Garland, The RPLG Group, P. O. Box 90796, Lakeland, Florida 33804-0796; (813) 688-8324. Psychotherapist specializing in reproductive (infertility and perinatal) and attachment issues and loss.

Stanislav and Christina Grof. Spiritual Emergence Network, 5905 Soquel Drive #650, Soquel, California 95073; or Association for Transpersonal Psychology, P. O. Box 4437, Stanford, California 94305. Courses in holotropic therapy, helping people heal themselves through reexperiencing preverbal events. Their techniques include holotropic breath work and evocative music, and are described in their book *The Adventure of Self-Discovery*.

Dawn J. Guzeman. 7761 Orangewood Avenue, Stanton, California 90680; (714) 892-7230. Experiential therapist for early childhood, prenatal, and past-life memories.

Rev. S. Vimala Infantino. 52555 Lanier Lane, Cumming, Georgia 30130; (404) 781-9412. Apprentice midwifery program for "Purebirth/Water birth." Monthly publication, *The Alliance Journal.* Counseling and natural healing. Dolphin water play with parents, newborns, and children.

Michael Irving. 274 Rhodes Avenue, Toronto, Ontario, Canada M4L 3A3; (416) 469-4764. Sculptor and primal therapist offering natalism workshop, "The Embryo Show," and healing birth and prenatal memories with art.

Phyllis Klaus. 1351 Arch Street, Berkeley, California 94708; (415) 528-1525. Marriage, family, and child counselor offering telephone counseling and hypnosis, expecially concerning birth issues.

Leah La Goy, 713 Peralta, Berkeley, California 94707; (510) 327-1521. Pre- and perinatal psychotherapy for infants, children and adults. Also therapy for the surviving twin.

Carista Luminaire, M.A., and John Mini, M.S.C.M., C.L.A. P. O. Box 633, Fairfax, California 94978; (415) 457-4942. Counseling, workshops and classes for holistic preconception and prenatal care in conscious conception, pregnancy, and childbirth.

Lisbeth Marcher and Erik Jarlness. BODYnamic Institute, 965 Talbot Street, Albany, California 94706; (415) 526-5201; and Schleppegrellsgade 7, 2200 Kebenhavn N, Denmark. Body-oriented psychotherapists.

Gayle Peterson, Ph.D. 1749 Vine Street, Berkeley, California 94703; (510) 526-5951. Preparation for childbirth, using the Peterson method of assessment and body-centered hypnosis for improving delivery outcome.

Eva Reich, M.D. P. O. Box 51, Hancock, Maine 04640; (207) 422-3122. World lecturer and leader of workshops in the use of bioenergetics, in particular for mothers and infants and health-care professionals.

Hanspeter Ruch, Ph.D. Gruzenstrasse 28, 8400 Winterthur, Switzerland; (052) 226-077. Primal therapist.

John-Richard and Troye Turner. Institute for Whole Self Discovery, Inc., Waterrod 92, 1613 CR Grootebroek, Netherlands; (31) 2285-13630. Prebirth therapists offering lectures, workshops, and private therapy sessions based on the prebirth analysis matrix.

Thomas R. Verny, M.D. 36 Madison Avenue, Toronto, Ontario, Canada M5R 2S1; (416) 929-5051. Psychiatrist offering individual and couples psychotherapy. Prenatal, preconception, adoption, and abortion counseling.

Joanna Wilheim. Rua Bocaina 81, São Paulo 05013, Brazil; (011) 650-833. Psychoanalyst also training therapists in working with pre- and perinatal matrices.

ORGANIZATIONS

American Academy of Medical Hypnosis Analysts. (AAMH) 710 East Ogden, Suite 208 Naperville, Illinois 60563; 1-(800)-34-HYPNO. Referrals to a range of health care practitioners with hypnoanalytic skills.

American Society of Clinical Hypnosis. 2200 E. Devon Ave., Suite 291, Des Plaines, Illinois 60018-4534; (708) 297-3317. Referrals to a variety of health care providers with doctoral degrees who use hypnosis.

Association for Transpersonal Psychology. P. O. Box 3049, Stanford, California 94309; (415) 327-2066. Quarterly Journal. (Box 4437). Annual conference, resources, and referrals to transpersonal therapists.

Association for Past-Life Research and Therapy. P. O. Box 20151, Riverside, California 92516; (714) 780-1030. Organized in 1980 to promote research and education in the field of regression or past-life therapy.

ATTACh (Association for Treatment and Training in the Attachment of Children). 2775 Villa Creek, Suite 240, Dallas, Texas 75234; (214) 247-2329.

Center for Sexual Abuse Counseling. 214 Market Street #14, Brighton, Massachusetts 02135; (617) 782-7664. Resources for adults who were sexually abused as children.

Institute for Bioenergetic Analysis. Alexander Lowen, M.D. 144 East 36th Street, New York, New York 10016; (212) 532-7742. A disciple of Wilhelm Reich, Lowen is the author of many books on bioenergetics and offers therapy and training sessions. He emphasizes a process of self-discovery using different, often stressful, postures designed to force the client's awareness of his or her character.

Institute for Cove Energetics, 115 East 23rd Street, New York, New York 10010; (212) 505-6767. Workshops, conferences, training, and research.

Institute for Shamanic Studies, Box 670m Belden Station, Norwalk, Connecticut 06852; (203) 454-2825. Workshops, resources, and referrals for Shamanic exploration and healing.

International Society of Prenatal and Perinatal Psychology and Medicine (ISPPM). Peter Fedor-Freybergh, M.D., Ph.D. Engelbrektsgatan 19, S-11432 Stockholm, Sweden. Founded in Europe in 1971, holds congresses every three years and publishes quarterly, *International Journal of Prenatal and Perinatal Studies*. Mattes Verlag GmbH, Postfach 103866 D-6900 Heidelberg, Germany.

International Society for the Research and Development of Haptonomy. Mas Del Ore, 66400 Oms, Ceret, France. Founded by Frans Veldman, haptonomy is the "science of touch and affectivity." Training courses offered for professionals in basic haptonomy, hapto-obstetrics, and hapto-psychotherapy.

International Primal Association (IPA). 2742 Fernwood Avenue, Roslyn, Pennsylvania 19001; (215) 887-9168. Resources, referrals, quarterly journal *Aesthema*.

Loving Relationships Training. 145 West 87 Street, New York, New York 10024; (212) 799-7323. Sondra Ray and Bob Mandel, founders. This process includes exploration of the effect of one's birth on choice of mate, and on the formation of a "personal law for life."

Pocket Ranch. 3960 West Sausal Lane, Healdsburg, California 95448; (707) 431-1516. Social worker and primal therapist Barbara Findeisen, director. A residential crisis center and therapy program situated in the mountains. Pre-, perinatal, and transpersonally oriented workshops.

Pre and Perinatal Psychology Association of North America (PPPANA). 1600 Prince St, #509, Alexandria, VA 22314. An educational nonprofit organization dedicated to the in-depth exploration of the psychological dimension of human reproduction and pregnancy, and the mental and emotional development of the unborn and newborn child. Members are professional and lay. PPPANA was founded in 1983 by Thomas Verny, M.D. It holds international conferences every two years and publishes the *Pre- and Perinatal Psychology Journal* four times annually. Verny edited the proceedings of the first congress in *Pre- and Perinatal Psychology: An Intro-duction* (New York: Human Sciences Press, 1987).

Radix Institute. P. O. Box 97, Ojai, California 93023; (805) 646-8555. Neo-Reichian psychologist Charles Kelley, Ph.D., established Radix training—"education in feeling and purpose." A unique feature of Radix programs is the emphasis on visual awareness, eye contact, seeing and being seen, and visualization techniques.

Spiritual Emergence Network (SEN). 5905 Soquel Drive #650, Soquel, California 95073; (408) 464-8261. Assistance, ed-ucation and research, referrals, and support for people undergoing nonordinary experiences—a "spiritual emer-gency" which often arises in conjunction with deep regressive psychotherapy.

Village Psychotherapy Group. 160 Bleecker Street, 9c East, New York, New York 10012; (212) 673-4618. Group practice of primal therapists in Greenwich Village.

GENERAL

American Gentle Birthing Association. 1804 S.W. Oak Knoll Court, Lake Oswego, Oregon 97034; (503) 636-7823. Mul-tidisciplinary group of physicians, health-care practitioners, birthing teachers, counselors, midwives, and infant massage instructors committed to gentle birthing.

American Society of Dowsers. Danville, Vermont 05828-0024; (802) 684-3417. Educational and scientific society open to all interested persons. Publishes the quarterly *American Dowser* and holds annual and regional conferences. Local chapters throughout the United States and liaisons with dowsers abroad.. Has bookstore and supply division.

Association for Research and Enlightenment (ARE). Edgar Cayce Foundation, P. O. Box 595, Virginia Beach, Virginia 23451; 1-(800) 368-2727. Organization for spiritual growth based on Edgar Cayce readings. Bimonthly journal *Venture Inward*, local study groups, regional conferences. ARE Medical Clinic, founded by William and Gladys McGarey, M.D.'s, 4018 North 40th Street, Phoenix, Arizona 85018, also practices healing advice recommended by Cayce. Holds residential personal-growth programs.

Centre Tomatis. 68 Boul. de Courcelles, 75017 Paris, France. Dr. Alfred Tomatis developed an "electronic ear," which screens out higher frequencies in a mother's voice so that it sounds like it would from inside the womb. This had been used to repair prenatal deprivation.

Circumcision Resource Center. Ronald Goldman, Director. Box 232, Boston, Massachusetts 02133; (617) 523-0088. Publications, support groups, lectures, and seminars to address the harm caused by circumcision.

Cunningham-Copia Foundation International Birth Project. P. O. Box 161113, Austin, Texas, 78716; (512) 327-8310. Resources for water birth, dolphin interaction, and training for birth facilitators.

Infant Development Education Association (IDSE). Catherine Thompson, President. 112 Braehead Drive, Fredericksburg, Virginia 22401; (703) 899-1565. Provides educational materials, instructors, certification in infant development techniques for prenatal, newborn, and infancy periods.

Infant-Parent Institute. Michael Trout, Director. 328 North Neil Street, Champaign, Illinois 61820; (217) 353-4060.

Private teaching and clinical service institute specializing in the problems of attachment in infants and adults.

Institute of Psychohistory. P. O. Box 401, New York, New York 10014-4397; (212) 873-5900. Resources, referrals, conferences, and quarterly journal edited by Lloyd deMause (my favorite periodical).

International Association of Infant Massage Instructors (IAIMI). 2350 Bowen Road, P. O. Box 438, Elma, New York 14059-0438; (716) 652-9789. Resources, referrals, and training of parents and professionals in nurturing touch.

International Awareness Network (ICAN). P. O. Box 152, Syracuse, New York 13210; (315) 424-1942. Activist organization with newsletter and seminars to help women avoid Cesareans and achieve vaginal birth after Cesareans (VBAC).

National Association for Perinatal Research and Education (NAPARE). 11 E. Hubbard Street, Suite 200, Chicago, Illinois 60611; (312) 329-2512. Treatment and study of drug-exposed children and educational programs.

National Organization of Circumcision Information Resources Centers (NOCIRC). P. O. Box 2512, San Anselmo, California 94979-2512; (415) 488-9883. Information, conferences, newsletter, book orders.

Michel Odent, M.D. 59 Roderick Road, London, NW3 2NP, U.K; (071) 485-0095; FAX (071) 267-5123. International birth attendant. "Last resource for women who cannot find anyone else." Lectures and workshops on birth, sexuality.

Prelearning Inc. Cedar Business Park, 15337 Northeast 92nd, Redmond, Washington 98052; 1-(800) 322-0859, ext. 100. Psychologist Brent Logan, Ph.D., developed a prelearning program using the "cardiac curriculum." A cassette player strapped to the pregnant belly delivers sixteen increasingly complex tapes to be played for an hour twice a week, starting at the sixth month.

Prenatal Classroom. Rene Van de Carr, M.D. 27255 Calaroga Avenue, Hayword, California 94545; "Prenatal Classroom" course to respond to a baby's kicks around the fifth month of pregnancy by poking back. At seven months, words are introduced with experiences, such as patting, stroking, rubbing, and shaking.

Touch Research Institute. Mailman Center for Child Development, University of Miami School of Medicine, P. O. Box 016820, Miami, Florida 33101. Sponsors professional education and research programs on the effects of various forms of therapeutic touch on human massage and disease.

Twinless Twin Support Group International, % Raymond Brandt, Ph. D. 11220 St. Joe Road, Ft. Wayne, Indiana 46835; (219) 627-5414. Networking, counseling, resources, quarterly newsletters.

Waterbirth International (a project of the Global Maternal/Child Health Association). Barbara Harper, R.N., Director. P. O. Box 366, West Linn, OR 97068; (503) 638-2930; FAX (805) 638-3634. Resources and referrals for water labor and water birth. Portable tubs are available and can be shipped anywhere in the world.

Women-to-Women. 1 Pleasant Street, Yarmouth, Maine 04096; (207) 846-6163. Physician-nurse practice with Christiane Northrup, M.D., past president of the American Holistic Medical Association. Emphasis on holistic counseling for wellness and therapy for abuse.

VIDEOTAPES

The Awakening and Growth of the Human: Studies in Infant Mental Health. Michael Trout. #1. "The Nature of Human Attachments in Infancy." #2, "The Psychological Dimensions of Pregnancy and Delivery." #3, "Conducting an Infant Mental Health Family Assessment." #4, "The Newborn, the Family and the Dance." #5, "The Birth of a Sick or Handicapped Baby: Impact on the Family." Additional videos on family events. Infant-Parent Institute, 328 N. Neil Street, Champaign, Illinois 61901; (217) 352-4060.

BabyJoy: Exercises and Activities for Parents and Newborns.

Elizabeth Noble and Leo Sorger. 448 Pleasant Lake Avenue, Harwich, Massachusetts 02645. Also includes massage, ball activities and aquatics with Carsten Noble Sorger.

The Birth Disc: A Visual Experience. A visual database of 9,000 photographs illustrating birth by Harriette Hartigan, presented in 65 chapters and 43 case studies. Image Premastering Services Ltd, 1781 Prior Avenue North, St. Paul, MN 55113; (612) 644-7802.

Channel for a New Life. Underwater birth of Carsten Sorger. Elizabeth Noble and Leo Sorger. 448 Pleasant Lake Avenue, Harwich, Massachusetts 02645. Spontaneous birth outdoors in a hot tub. Shows squatting position and much vocalization. A video about trusting and surrendering to the forces of Nature.

Childbirth at a Turning Point: Michel Odent. Crystal Visions Association. 6289 Westmoreland Place, Goleta, California 03117. Videotaped seminar with this famous French obstetrician discussing his theories of labor and birth.

A Gift for Unborn Children. Bradley Boatman Productions. 33246 Pacific Coast Highway, Malibu, California 90265; (213) 457-2884. Explores fetal development and emphasizes prenatal bonding and natural childbirth. Interviews with prominent pre- and perinatal psychologists.

Journey to Be Born. Barbara Findeisen. 3960 W. Sausal Lane, Healdsburg, California 95448; (707) 431-1516. Excellent introduction to regression experiences pre- and perinatal psychology. Interview with experts and clients, and critiques of interventive birth practices.

Knowing the Unborn: Pre-Birth Parenting. A 29-minute video on emotional bonding with the unborn. Royda and Kelley Ballard. 2554 Lincoln Boulevard, #509, Marina del Rey, California 90291; (213) 417-3663.

Long Ago Hurt. A 35mm film about the trauma of birth and womb life, and a group of people who were able to reach a deeper understanding of their life by reliving those early experiences. P. O. Box 303 Camberwell, Victoria 3124, Australia.

The Miracle of Life. Lennart, Nilsson, Boston: WGBH Educational Foundation, 1983. Magnificent photography of human development from conception to birth.

Touch The Future. Mendizza and Associates. 4350 Lime Avenue, Long Beach, California 90807; (213) 426-2627. A video project for social transformation based on pre- and perinatal research, via mass media.

Waterbabies. Video documentary on water birth. Point of View Productions, 2477 Folsom Street, San Francisco, California 94110; (415) 821-0435.

AUDIOCASSETTES

The Child Within. Leni Schwartz, 197 Oakdale, Mill Valley, California 94941. Guided meditations for expectant parents.

Healing Your Prenatal Memories. Clara Riley, Mother/Fetus Communication, 31542 Coast Highway, Suite 2, South Laguna, California 92677.

Inside Experiences: Guided Recall of Birth and Before. Elizabeth Noble, 448 Pleasant Lake Avenue, Harwich, Massachusetts 02645; (508) 432-8040; FAX (508) 432-9685. Appendix I in various languages set to specially composed music.

Heartsongs. Leon Thurman and Anna Peters Langness, Music Study Services, P. O. Box 4665, Englewood, Colorado 80155. Music for the unborn child and newborn.

Journey into Parenting. Two-cassette exploration for couples to enchance preconception bonding. P. O. Box 633, Fairfax, California 94978; (415) 457-4942.

Prelearning Inc. Cedar Business Park, 15337 Northeast 92nd, Redmond, Washington 98052; 1-(800) 322-0859, ext. 100. Psychologist Brent Logan, Ph.D., developed a prelearning program using the "cardiac curriculum." A cassette player strapped to the pregnant belly delivers sixteen increasingly complex tapes to be played for an hour twice a day per week, starting at the sixth month.

Love Chords. Thomas Verny and Sandra Collier, A & M Records of Canada, Scarborough, Ontario, Canada. Classical music for the unborn and newborn.

Lullaby from the Womb. Hajime Murooka, M.D., Capitol Records, Hollywood, California. Heartbeat sounds superimposed on classical music.

Music for Bonding. Royda and Kelley Ballard, 2554 Lincoln Boulevard, #509, Marina del Rey, California 90291; (213) 417-3663. (800) 772-1172.

Transitions: Womb Sounds. Natural harmonies for mother and child; soothing music for crying infants. Placenta Music Inc, 2675 Acorn Avenue NE, Atlanta, Georgia 30305; (404) 262-1559.

Relax and Enjoy Your Baby Within. Sylvia Klein Olkin. Relaxation and visualization set to music. Be Healthy Inc. 51 Salrock Road, Baltic, Connecticut, 06330 (800) 433-5523.

Bibliography & Further Reading

BOOKS

Aivanhov, Master Omraam Mikhael. *Education Begins before Birth*. Los Angeles: Editions Prosveta, 1982.

―――. *The Splendour of Tipheret*. Los Angeles: Editions Prosveta, 1977.

―――. *Hope for the World: Spiritual Galvanoplasty*. Los Angeles: Editions Prosveta, 1984.

Apley, John. *The Child with Abdominal Pain*. 2nd ed. London: Blackwell, 1975.

Avery, Jeanne. *Astrology and Your Past Lives*. New York: Simon & Schuster, 1987.

Arditti, Rita, et al. *Test-tube Women: What Future for Motherhood?* Boston: Pandora Press, 1984.

Bach, Edward. *Heal Thyself: An Explanation of the Real Cause and Cure of Disease*. Saffron Walden, Essex, U.K.: C. W. Daniel Company Ltd., 1931.

Bailey, Alice. *Treatise on Cosmic Fire*. New York: Lucis, 1951.

Baker, Jeannine Parvati. *Conscious Conception: Elemental Journey Through the Labyrinth of Sexuality*. Monroe, UT: Freestone, 1986.

————. *Hygieia: A Woman's Herbal.* Monroe, UT: Freestone, 1978.

————. *Prenatal Yoga and Natural Birth.* Monroe, UT: Freestone, 1986.

Bettelheim, Bruno. *The Uses of Enchantment.* London: Penguin, 1975.

Boadella, David, ed. *In the Wake of Reich.* London: Coventure, 1976.

————. *Lifestreams: An Introduction to Biosynthesis.* New York: Routledge and Kegan Paul, 1987.

Borysenko, Joan. *Minding the Body; Mending the Mind.* Reading, MA: Addison-Wesley, 1987.

Brenner, Paul. *Health Is a Question of Balance.* Marina Del Rey, CA: DeVorss & Co., 1978.

————. *Life Is a Shared Creation.* Marina Del Rey, CA: DeVorss & Co., 1981.

Briggs, Dorothy C. *Your Child's Self-Esteem: The Key to His Life.* New York: Doubleday, 1977.

Campbell, Joseph, and Bill Moyers. *The Power of Myth.* New York: Doubleday, 1988.

Capra, Fritjof. *The Tao of Physics.* New York: Bantam, 1975.

Carson, Anne, ed. *Spiritual Parenting in the New Age.* Freedom, CA: Crossing Press, 1989.

Chamberlain, David. *Babies Remember Birth.* Los Angeles: Tarcher, 1988.

Chicago, Judy. *The Birth Project.* New York: Doubleday, 1985.

Church, Dawson. *Communicating with the Spirit of Your Unborn Child.* San Leandro, CA: Aslan Publishing, 1988.

Cohen, Nancy Wainer. *Open Season: Survival Guide for Natural Childbirth and VBAC in the 90s.* New York: Bergin and Garvey, 1991.

Corda, Murshida Vera Justin. *Cradle of Heaven: Psychological and Spiritual Dimensions of Conception, Pregnancy and Birth.* Lebanon Springs, NY: Omega Press, 1987.

Crookhall, Robert. *Out of Body Experiences.* New York: Ballantine, 1980.

DeMause, Lloyd. *Foundations of Psychohistory.* New York: Creative Books, 1982.

DeRohan, Ceanne. *The Right Use of Will: Healing and Evolving the Emotional Body*. Albuquerque: One World Publications, 1984.

Diamond, John. *The Re-Mothering Experience*. Valley Cottage, NY: Archaeus Press, 1981.

————. *The Body Doesn't Lie*. New York: Warner, 1979.

————. *Speech, Language and the Power of Breath*. Valley Cottage, NY: Archaeus Press, 1979.

————. *Behavorial Kinesiology*. New York: Harper and Row, 1979.

————. *The Collected Papers of John Diamond, M.D.* Vol. II. Valley Cottage, NY: Archaeus Press, 1980.

————. *Life Energy*. New York: Dodd Mead & Co., 1985.

————. *Life Energy Analysis: A Way to Cantillation*. Valley Cottage, NY: Archaeus Press, 1988.

Dossey, Larry. *Space, Time and Medicine*. Boulder, CO: Shambhala, 1982.

Dublin, L. and B. Bunzel. *To Be or Not to Be: A Study of Suicide*. New York: Quinn & Oden, 1933.

Earnshaw, Avril. *Family Time*. Sydney: A & K Enterprises, 1983.

Emerson, William. *Infant and Childbirth Refacilitation*. Guildford, U.K.: University of Surrey Press, 1984.

————. *Infant Birth Refacilitation: A Film*. Petaluma, CA: Human Potential Resources, 1986.

————. *Implosive Containment in Infant Primal Therapy*. Petaluma, CA: Human Potential Resources, 1986.

English, Jane. *Different Doorway: Adventures of a Cesarean Born*. Mt. Shasta, CA: Earth Heart, 1985.

Fedor-Freybergh, Peter G. & M. L. Vanessa Vagel, eds. *Prenatal and Perinatal Psychology and Medicine: Encounter with the Unborn*. Park Ridge, NJ: Parthenon, 1988.

Feher, Leslie. *The Psychology of Birth*. New York: Continuum, 1981.

Feldmar, Andrew. "The Embryology of Consciousness: What Is a normal pregnancy? In *The Psychological Aspects of Abortion*, D. Mall and W. Watts, eds. Washington, DC: University Publications of America, 1979.

Findlay, Arthur. *On the Edge of the Etheric*. London: Psychic Press, 1931.

Fodor, Nandor. *In Search of the Beloved: A Clinical Investigation of the Trauma of Birth and Prenatal Conditioning*. New York: Hermitage, 1949.

Freud, Sigmund. *The Problem of Anxiety*. New York: Norton, 1936.

Gabriel, Michael. *Voices From the Womb*. Lower Lake, California: Aslan Publishing, 1992.

Gawain, Shakki. *Living in the Light*. San Rafael, CA: New World Library, 1986.

Gazzaniga, Michael S. *Mind Matters—How the Mind and Brain Interact to Create Our Conscious Lives*. Boston: Houghton Mifflin, 1989.

Grandin, Temple and Margaret M. Scariano. *Emergence: Labelled Autistic*. Novato, California: Arena Press, 1986.

Greer, Germaine. *Sex and Destiny: The Politics of Fertility*. London: Pan, 1985.

Grobstein, Clifford. *Science and the Unborn*. New York: Basic Books, 1988.

Groddeck, Georg. *The Book of the It*. London: C. W. Daniel, 1935; New York: Vintage, 1949 (first published in German in 1923).

Grof, Stanislav. *Realms of the Human Unconscious*. New York: Dutton, 1976.

———. *The Adventure of Self-Discovery*. Albany: SUNY Press, 1988.

———. *Beyond the Brain: Birth, Death and Transcendence in Psychotherapy*. Albany: SUNY Press, 1985.

Hay, Louise. *Heal Your Body*. Santa Monica, CA: Hay House, 1988.

Hodson, Geoffrey. *The Miracle of Birth: A Clairvoyant Study of a Human Embryo*. Wheaton, IL: Theosophical Publishing House, 1981.

Holt, John. *Teach Your Own*. New York: Delta, 1981.

Janov, Arthur. *The Primal Scream*. New York: Putnam, 1970.

———. *Imprints*. New York: Coward McCann, 1983.

————. *The Feeling Child*. New York: Simon & Schuster, 1973.

Johnsen, Lillemor. *Integrated Respiration Theory/Therapy: Birth and Rebirth in the Fullness of Time*. International Institute for Respiration Therapy, Bergsliengate 6, 0342 Oslo, Norway, 1981.

Johnson, Sonia. *Going Out of Our Minds: The Metaphysics of Liberation*. Freedom, CA: Crossing Press, 1987.

Jung, Carl G., ed. *Man and His Symbols*. New York: Dell, 1964

Kahn, Sufi Inayat. *Education from Birth to Maturity*. Geneva, Switzerland: Sufi Publishing Company, 1974.

Keleman, Stanley. *Emotional Anatomy*. Berkeley: Center Press, 1985.

————. *Your Body Speaks Its Mind*. Berkeley: Center Press, 1981.

Kennell, John and Marshall Klaus. *Parent-Infant Bonding*. St. Louis: Mosby, 1982.

Klaus, Marshall and Phyllis. *The Amazing Newborn: Discovering and Enjoying Your Baby's Natural Abilities*. Reading, MA: Addison-Wesley, 1985.

Klimek, Rudolf, ed. *Pre- and Perinatal Psycho-Medicine*. Cracow: DWN DReAM, 1992.

Laing, Ronald D. *The Facts of Life*. New York: Ballantine, 1976.

————. *The Divided Self*. New York: Penguin, 1965.

————. *The Voice of Experience*. New York: Pantheon, 1982.

————. *Knots*. New York: Penguin, 1970.

Lake, Frank. *Studies in Constricted Confusion: Exploration of a Pre- and Peri-natal Paradigm*. Nottingham, U.K.: Clinical Theology Association. St. Mary's House, Church Westcote, Oxford OX76SF, England, 1981.

————. *Clinical Theology*. New York: Crossroad, 1987.

————. *Tight Corners in Pastoral Counseling*. London: Darton, Longman and Todd, 1981.

Landsman, Sandra G. *Found: A Place For Me*. Jupiter, FL: Treehouse Enterprises, 1984.

————. *I'm Special: An Experiential Workbook for the Child In Us All*, Jupiter, FL: Treehouse Enterprises, 1986.

LeBoyer, Frederick. *Birth Without Violence*. New York: Knopf, 1975.

Levine, Stephen. *Who Dies? A Manual for Conscious Living and Conscious Dying*. New York: Doubleday, 1982.

Lowen, Alexander. *Bioenergetics*. New York: Penguin, 1975.

————. *Depression and the Body: The Biological Basis of Faith and Reality*. New York: Penguin, 1973.

Mackarness, Richard. *Not All in the Mind*. London: Pan, 1976.

MacNutt, Francis and Judith. *Praying for Your Unborn Child*. New York: Doubleday, 1988.

Maher, J. M., and Dennie Briggs. *An Open Life: Joseph Campbell in conversation with Michael Toms*. Burdett, NY: Larson, 1988.

Marnie, Eve. *Love Start: Pre-Birth Bonding*. Santa Monica, CA: Hay House, 1989.

Marrone, Robert. *Body of Knowledge*. Albany, NY: SUNY Press, 1990.

May, Rollo. *The Discovery of Being: Writings in Existential Psychology*. New York: Norton, 1986.

McGarey, Gladys. *Born to Live*. Phoenix, AZ: Gabriel Press, 1980.

McGoldrick, M., and Gzerso, R. *Genograms in Family Assessment*. New York: Norton, 1985.

Meher Baba. *Listen, Humanity*. Narrated and edited by D. E. Stevens. New York: Harper and Row.

Millar, Christopher J. *The First Act of Life*. 1984.

————. *Matters of Life and Birth: A Personal Perspective on Primal Therapy*. Creswick, Aust., 1981.

Montagu, Ashley. *Touching: The Human Significance of the Skin*. New York: Harper and Row, 1986.

————. *Life Before Birth*. New York: NAL, 1965.

————. *Prenatal Influences*. Springfield, IL: CC Thomas, 1962.

Moody, Raymond A. Jr. *Life after Life*. New York: Dutton, 1976.

————. *The Light Beyond*. New York: Bantam, 1988.

Mott, Francis. *The Nature of the Self*. London: Allen Wingate, 1959.

————. *The Universal Design of Birth*. Philadelphia: David McKay, 1952.

————. *A Child Is Born*. New York: Delacorte, 1990.

Noble, Elizabeth. *Essential Exercises for the Childbearing Year*. Boston: Houghton Mifflin, 1988.

————. *Having Twins*. Rev. ed. Boston: Houghton Mifflin, 1991.

————. *Childbirth with Insight*. Boston: Houghton Mifflin, 1983.

————. *Having Your Baby by Donor Insemination*. Boston: Houghton Mifflin, 1988.

Odent, Michel. *Birth Reborn*. New York: Pantheon, 1984.

————. *Primal Health: A Blueprint for Our Survival*. London: Century, 1986.

————. *Entering the World*. New York: NAL, 1984.

Orr, Leonard, and Sondra Ray. *Rebirthing in the New Age*. Berkeley: Celestial Arts, 1975.

Pearce, Joseph Chilton. *The Crack in the Cosmic Egg: Challenging Constructs of Mind and Reality*. New York: Crown, 1988.

————. *Exploring the Crack in the Cosmic Egg*. New York: Pocketbooks, 1982.

————. *Magical Child*. New York: Bantam, 1981.

————. *Magical Child Matures*. New York: Bantam, 1986.

Peerbolte, M. Lietaert. *Prenatal Dynamics*. Leyden, Netherlands: Uitgeverij Sijthoff, 1954.

Peterson, Gayle. *Birthing Normally*. Berkeley: Mindbody Press, 1981.

————. *An Easier Childbirth*. Los Angeles: Tarcher, 1991.

Peterson, Gayle, and Lewis Mehl. *Pregnancy as Healing*. Vol. I and II. Berkeley: Mindbody Press, 1984.

Pierrakos, John. *Core Energetics*. Mendocino, CA: LifeRhythm, 1990.

Radhakrishnan, S. *The Cultural Heritage of India*. Calcutta: University Press, 1958.

Rank, Otto. *The Trauma of Birth*. London: Routledge, 1929.

Ray, Sondra, and Bo Mandel. *Birth and Relationships*. Berkeley: Celestial Arts, 1987.

Ridgway, Roy. *The Unborn Child: How To Recognize and Over-*

come Prenatal Trauma. Aldershot, Harts UK: Wildwood, 1987.

Reich, Wilhelm. Children of the Future. New York: Farrar, Straus & Giroux, 1983.

———. The Function of the Orgasm. New York: Simon & Schuster, 1973.

———. Character Analysis. New York: Farrar, Straus & Giroux, 1969.

Ribble, Margaret. The Rights of Infants. New York: Columbia University Press, 1943.

Ring, Kenneth. Heading Toward Omego: The Near Death Experience and Human Evolution. New York: Morrow, 1984.

Rossi, Ernest L., and David B. Cheek. Mind-Body Therapy: Methods of Ideodynamic Healing in Hypnosis. New York: Norton, 1988.

Rothman, Barbara K. The Tentative Pregnancy: Women's Experiences of Amniocentesis. New York: Viking, 1986.

Ruch, Hanspeter. The Experience of Being Born as Recalled in Adulthood. Ph.D. Thesis, Lesley College, Cambridge, MA, 1985.

Sabom, Michael. Recollections of Death. New York: Harper and Row, 1981.

Saint-Pierre, Gaston and Debbie Boater. The Metamorphic Technique. York Beach, ME: Samuel Weiser, 1982.

Schwartz, Leni. The World of the Unborn. New York: Richard Marek, 1980.

Sheldrake, Rupert. The Presence of the Past. New York: Time-Life, 1988.

Siegel, Bernie. Love, Medicine and Miracles. New York: Harper and Row, 1986.

———. Peace, Love and Healing: Body/Mind Communication and the Path to Self Healing. New York: Harper and Row, 1990.

Solter, Aletha J. The Aware Baby. Goleta, CA: Shining Star, 1984.

Star, Rima Beth. The Healing Power of Birth. Austin, TX: Star Publishing, 1986.

Steadman, Alice. *Who's the Matter with Me*. Marina Del Rey, CA: DeVorss & Co., 1977.

Thich Nhat Hanh. *Being Peace*. Berkeley: Parallax, 1987.

Tomatis, Alfred A. *La Nuit Uterine*. Paris: Editions Stock, 1981.

Tompkins, Peter and Christopher Bird. *The Secret Life of Plants*. New York: Harper and Row, 1989.

Tournier, Paul. *The Meaning of Persons*. London: SCM, 1957.

Turner, J.R. *Birth, Life and More Life*. Santa Fe, New Mexico: Whole Self Publishing, 1989.

Veldman, Frans. *L'Haptonomie*. Paris: PUF, 1988.

Verny, Thomas R., and John Kelly. *The Secret Life of the Unborn Child*. New York: Summit, 1981.

————, ed. *Pre- and Peri-natal Psychology: An Introduction*. New York: Human Sciences Press, 1987.

————. *Parenting Your Unborn Child*. Toronto: Doubleday, 1988.

Vlcek, J. *Journey into the World: My Life Before Birth*. Don Mills, Ontario: Elf Publishing, 1989.

Waring, Marilyn. *If Women Counted*. San Francisco: Harper and Row, 1989.

Watts, Alan. *The Wisdom of Insecurity*. New York: Random House, 1970.

Weiss, Brian. *Many Lives, Many Masters*. New York: Simon & Schuster, 1988.

————. *Through Time into Healing*. New York: Simon & Schuster, 1992.

Wilson Schaef, Anne. *When Society Becomes an Addict: Meditations for Women Who Do Too Much*. New York: Harper and Row, 1990.

Winnicott, D. W. "Birth Memories, Birth Trauma and Anxiety." In *Through Pediatrics to Psychoanalysis: Collected Papers*. New York: Basic Books, 1958.

Woodward, Mary Anne. *Scars of the Soul: Holistic Healing in the Edgar Cayce Readings*. Fair Grove, MO: Brindabella Books, 1985.

ARTICLES

Blasband, Richard A., et al. "Muscular Armoring in Labor: An Orgonomic (Bioenergetic) Perspective." *Pre- and Perinatal Psychology Journal* 6(1), Fall 1991.

Buchheimer, Arnold. "Memory: Preverbal and Verbal" in Verny T. R. ed. *Pre- and Perinatal Psychology: An Introduction.* New York: Human Sciences Press, 1987.

Cayce, Edgar. Readings available from the Association for Research and Enlightenment and the Edgar Cayce Foundation, P.O. Box 595 Virginia Beach, Virginia 23451 (804) 428-3588.

Chamberlain, David. "The Outer Limits of Memory." *Noetic Sciences Review*, Autumn 1990.

———. "Babies Remember Pain." *Pre- and Perinatal Psychology Journal* 3(4), Summer 1989.

———. "Reliability of Birth Memories: Evidence from Mother and Child Pairs in Hypnosis." *Journal of the American Academy of Medical Hypnoanalysts* 1(2), 1986: 89–98.

———. "The Cognitive Newborn: A Scientific Update." *British Journal of Psychotherapy* 4(1), 1987: 30–71.

———. "Is There Intelligence Before Birth?" *Pre- and Perinatal Psychology Journal* 6(3), 1992.

Cheek, David B. "Sequential Head and Shoulder Movements Appearing with Age Regression in Hypnosis to Birth." *American Journal of Clinical Hypnosis* 16(4), 1974: 261–66.

———. "Prenatal and Perinatal Imprints: Apparent Prenatal Consciousness as Revealed by Hypnosis." *Pre- and Perinatal Psychology Journal* 1(2), 1986: 109.

Colter, Marvin W., "Sexual Cross-identity as a Fetal Response to Subliminal Parent Messages." In Fedor-Freybergh, Peter G. & M. L. Vaness Vogel, eds., *Prenatal and Perinatal Psychology and Medicine: Encounter with the Unborn.* Park Ridge, NJ: Parthenon, 1988.

Croft-Long E. "The Placenta in Love and Legend", *Bulletin of the Medical Library Association* 51, 1963: 233–241.

Davidson, J. R. "The Shadow of Life: Psychosocial Explanations for Placental Rituals." *Culture, Medicine and Psychiatry* 9, 1985: 75–92.

Davis-Floyd, Robbie. "Hospital Birth Routines as Rituals: Society's Messages to American Women." *Pre- and Perinatal Psychology* 1(4), Summer 1987.

De Casper, A. and W. Fifer. "Of Human Bonding: Newborns Prefer Their Mother's Voices" *Science* 208, 1980: 1174–76.

deMause, Lloyd. "The Universality of Incest." *Journal of Psychohistory* 19(2), Spring 1992.

Dolto-Tolitch, Catherine. "Contribution of Perinatal Haptonomy to Children's Medicine." *Clinical Testimony* 21, 1988.

Dörner, Günter. "Significance of Hormones and Neurotransmitters in Pre- and Early Postnatal Life for Human Ontogenesis." *International Journal of Prenatal and Perinatal Studies* 1(2), 1989.

Dowling, Terence. "The Use of Placental Symbols in Psychotherapy." In *Prenatal Psychology and Medicine: Encounter with the Unborn*, Peter Fedor-Freybergh, ed. Carnforth, U.K.: Parthenon Publishing, 1988.

———. "The Significance of Pre- and Perinatal Experience in Child Psychotherapy." *International Journal of Prenatal and Perinatal Studies* 1(3), 1989.

———. "The Psychological Significance of the Fetal Skin Activity." *International Journal of Prenatal and Perinatal Studies* 2(2), June 1990.

Emerson, William. "Life, Birth and Rebirth: The Hazy Mirrors." *European Journal of Humanistic Psychology* 6, 1978.

Fodor, Nandor. "The Psychology of Numbers." *Journal of Clinical Psychopathology*, July–October 1947.

Freedman, D. G., F. H. Boerman, and N. Freedman. "Effects of Kinesthetic Stimulation on Weight Gain and Smiling in Premature Infants." *American Journal of Orthopsychiatry*, April 1960.

Gardner, S. L., K. R. Garland and S. Merenstein. "The Neonate and the Environment: Impact on Development." *Handbook of Neonatal Intensive Care* Chapter 24. St. Louis: Mosby, 1989.

Goldblatt, David B. "The Practical Application of Existential

Phenomenological Psychotherapy in a Residential Setting."
SEN Newsletter, Spring 1987.

Hall, Calvin S. "Prenatal and Birth Experiences in Dreams."
Psychoanalytic Review 54, 1967: 157–74.

Harary, Keith. "Womb with a View." *Omni*, August 1989.

Hårkansson, T. "Prenatal Memories." *International Journal of Prenatal and Perinatal Studies* 1(3), 1989.

Hull, William F. "Psychological Treatment of Birth Trauma with Age Regression and Its Relationship to Chemical Dependency." *Pre- and Perinatal Psychology* 1(2), Winter 1986.

Jacobsen, Bertil. "Perinatal Origin of Eventual Self-Destructive Behavior." *Pre- and Perinatal Psychology* 2(4), Summer 1988.

Janus, Ludwig. "The Hidden Dimension of Prenatal and Perinatal Experience in the Works of Freud, Jung, and Klein." *International Journal of Prenatal and Perinatal Studies* 1(1), March 1989.

———. "The Trauma of Birth as Reflected in the Psycho-Analytic Process." In *Prenatal and Perinatal Psychology: Encounter with the Unborn*, P. Fedor-Freybergh and M. I. Vogel, eds. Carnforth, UK: Parthenon, 1988.

Khamsi, Stephen. "Birth Feelings: A Phenomenological Investigation." *Aesthema* 7, January 1987.

Lagercrantz, Hugo, and Theodore A. Slotkin. "The 'Stress' of Being Born." *Scientific American* (254), April 1986: 100–107.

Laibow, R. E. "Prenatal and Perinatal Experience and Developmental Impairment." In *Prenatal and Perinatal Psychology and Medicine*, P. G. Fedor-Freybergh and M. L. Vogel, eds. Carnforth, U.K.: Parthenon, 1988.

Landsman, S. G. "Metaphors: The Language of Pre- and Perinatal Trauma" *Pre- and Perinatal Psychology* 4(1), Fall 1989.

Lifton, Robert Jay. "On Death and the Continuity of Life: A New Paradigm." *Journal of Psychohistory* 1(4), Spring 1974.

Liley, A. W. "The Foetus as a Personality." *Australian and New Zealand Journal of Psychiatry* 6(2), 1972: 99–105.

Laukaran, V. H., and B. J. Van den Borg. "The Relationship of Maternal Attitudes to Pregnancy Outcome and Obstetric

Complications: A Cohort Study of Unwanted Pregnancy." *American Journal of Obstetrical Gynecology* 126, 1980: 374.

Lawson, Alvin H. "Perinatal Imagery in UFO Abduction Reports." *Journal of Psychohistory* 12(2), Fall 1984.

Long, E. Croft. "The Placenta in Lore and Legend." *Bulletin Medical Library Association* 51, 1963: 233–241.

Marchesan, Rolando. "Age Regression in Hypnosis—Confirmed by the Handwriting, Tree and Family Tests." *International Journal of Prenatal and Perinatal Studies* 2(4), December 1990.

Mathison, Linda. "Does Your Child Remember?" *Mothering*, Fall 1981: 103–107.

Mehl, Lewis E. "Psychobiosocial Intervention in Threatened Premature Labor." *Pre- and Perinatal Psychology* 3(1), Fall 1988.

————. "Hypnosis and Prenatal Memory." *International Journal of Prenatal and Perinatal Studies* 1(4), 1989: 381–86.

Melzack, Ronald. "Phantom Limbs." *Scientific American*, April 1992: 266(4): 120–22

Moody, Raymond. "Beyond the Light." *Venture Inward* 7(2), March-April 1991: 12.

Ngakpa Chogyam Togden, Ven Lam. "Inner Tantra: Embracing Emotions as the Path." *SEN Newsletter*, Winter 1991.

"New Theory Links Schizophrenia to Problems in Corpuls Callosum." *Brain/Mind Bulletin* 15(6), March 1990.

Odent, Michel. "Children of the Future." *Resurgence* 132, January 1989.

Pert, Candace, et al. "Neuropeptides and Their Receptors: A Psychosomatic Network." *Journal of Immunology* 135(2) Supplement, 1985: 820–26.

Piontelli, Alessandra, "A Study on Twins Before and After Birth." *Int. Rev. Psycho-Anal.* 16, 1989: 413–426.

Pribran, Karl H. "The Cognitive Revolution in Brain Issues." *American Psychologist* 41(5), 1986: 507–20.

Raikov, V. L. "Age Regression to Infancy by Adult Subjects in Deep Hypnosis" *American Journal of Clinical Hypnosis* 22, 1980: 156–163.

Riley, Clara. "Transuterine Communication in Problem Pregnancies." *Pre- & Perinatal Psychology Journal*, 1(3) 1987: 180–190.

Sadger, J. "Sleep Walking and Moon Walking." *Nervous and Mental Disease Monograph Series* 31, 1920.

———. "Preliminary Study of the Psychic Life of the Fetus and the Primary Germ." *Psychoanalytic Review*, July 1941.

Salk, Lee. "Thoughts on the Concept of Imprinting And its Place in Early Human Development." *Canadian Psychiatric Association Journal* 11, 1966: S296.

———. "Mother's Heartbeat as an Imprinting Stimulus." *Transcripts of the New York Academy of Science* 24, 1962: 752–63.

———. "Some Schizophrenia May Have Origins in Fetal or Perinatal Life." *Ob-Gyn News* 25(2), January 15–31, 1990.

———. et al. "Relationship of Maternal and Perinatal Conditions to Eventual Adolescent Suicide." *Lancet* 1, 1985: 624–27.

Seely, Stephen. "Do Dreams Make Sense?" *New Scientist*, May 1984, 17: 37–38.

Shevirin, H. and P. W. Toussieng. "Conflict Over Tactile Experiences in Emotionally Disturbed Children." *Journal American Academy of Child Psychiatry.* 1 (4): 564–590.

Silberer, Herbert. "Spermatozoenträume," and "Zur Frage der Spermatozoenträume." In *Jahrbuch Fur Psychoana Pytische Und Psychopathologische Forschungen.* IV.BAND, 1912.

Sontag, L. W. "Differences in Modifiability of Fetal Behavior and Physiology." *Psychosomatic Medicine* 6, 1944.

———. "Implications of Fetal Behavior and Environment for Adult Personalities." *Annals of the New York Academy of Sciences* 134, 1965: 782–6.

Stevenson, Ian. "American Children Who Claim to Remember Previous Lives." *Journal of Nervous and Mental Diseases* 171 (12): 742–48.

Tulving, Endel. "How Many Memory Systems Are There?" *American Psychologist* 40(4), 1985: 385–98.

"Unwanted Children Face Struggle." *Brain-Mind Bulletin* 15(2), November 1989.

Verrier, Nancy. "The Primal Wound: Understanding the Adopted Child." Paper presented at the Fourth International Congress on Pre- and Perinatal Psychology, Amherst, MA, August 1989.

Wallach, Edward. "Communication with the Fetus." *Contemporary OB/GYN* July 1988: 23–28.

Watkins, Helen. "Treating the Traumas of Abortion." *Pre- & Perinatal Psychology Journal* 1(2), 1986: 135–42.

Weintraub, Pamela. "Preschool?" *Omni*, August 1989.

Wile, I. S., and R. Davis. "The Relation of Birth to Behavior." *American Journal of Orthopsychiatry* 11, 1941: 330–34.

Index